Don't Call Me Mum!

Text copyright © 2012

All Rights Reserved

This book is dedicated to:

All the family and friends who have supported me over the years.

All names have been changed

Don't Call Me Mum!

Foreword

"I blame the parents!"

Does this sound familiar? It does to me. The words resonate in my ears. "It's not *always* their fault!" I want to scream. "Some have tried everything!"

I, the mother of a son who has had convictions for thefts, drugs and criminal damage as well as being permanently excluded from school and ostracised from everyone we know, have attracted a multitude of comments from many holding the 'blame the parents' opinion.

What they don't know is that at the age of one-and-a-half, when he would not sleep, destroyed everything he laid his hands on, and threw Oscar-winning tantrums, I began trailing him to every available 'expert' in the field of child and adolescent behavioural problems.

Health Visitors blamed my separation from his father in infancy; the GP suspected maternal depression whilst 0-19 team conceded his conduct to be a result of my youth and inexperience.

Further down the line, child psychologists asserted his diet as a contributory factor, meanwhile child psychiatrists held *my* background responsible. Teachers delved into his home life, social services suspected abuse and the youth offending team attributed peer pressure. The police blamed *him* and the courts punished *me*.

Counting The Cost

I like lists. I create at least one every day. Sometimes, I jot down lists of what lists I need to write!

Today, I'm recording all the things my son has broken this year.

1. kettle
2. bathroom door
3. microwave
4. fridge freezer
5. play station control pad
6. play station
7. two mobile phones
8. numerous glasses, cups, etc
9. outside security light
10. drainpipe at front of house
11. drainpipe at back of house
12. cupboard door
13. hinges on bathroom window
14. two holes punched in wall;

I could list all the things he has stolen or sold too. But I'll come to that later.

Don't Call Me Mum!
My Problem

October 2009 (Aged 15 years, 9 months)

"Social Services are unlikely to do anything," she stated gently as I howled in anguish down the telephone.

"He can't come back here!" I paced the room as I stated my case. "We're going to lose our home because of him!" *I can't take it any more!*

I slowly replaced the receiver, sinking with it into the floor. Now my voice had stilled; the house was eerily quiet. All fight was slipping out of me. The plan had been to tell them straight.

Breaking point had been reached.

The teacher at the pupil referral unit, had listened patiently as I ranted, making all the right noises. Yet I detected an undercurrent of disbelief in her replies as though she thought I was exaggerating.

I suddenly caught sight of myself in the bedroom mirror. Lately, I seemed to be spending a lot of time in my room. Trying to escape his name calling, taunts and threats, not to mention the constant bullying for money I did not have and could not give. He was not choosy who he would then steal from to ensure his insatiable demands were met: family, friends, shops, neighbours or strangers.

The salty taste of my tears trickled over my lips as I observed my pallid reflection.

Was that really me?

I barely recognised myself anymore. Clad in baggy tracksuit bottoms and a shapeless jumper, I had become lost between the deepening lines on my face. Lines that should belong to a woman ten years my senior.

Night-after-night, I was becoming more depleted; awoken by his nocturnal homecomings or hooded associates. Instead of sleep, fear would stand guard. Unlike my son's degenerate 'friends' whose faceless existence brought security, my constant companion had two faces of fear. One face reflected uncertainty;

where he was, who he was with, whether he was ok. The other reflected hatred for the miserable life he was forcing me to lead.

    Anyway, this latest attempt at seeking help was as futile as all the previous ones I had made. He was nobody else's problem. Mine and mine alone.
    He did not reappear that day. The phone call I had made would have been made known to him. Maybe he felt ashamed at the disgusting names he had called me that morning. Or the threat to smash up my car. It took an eternity to drop off to sleep that night. As his mother, I was still forced to endure the usual images, which consisted of my worst fears intruding into my shattered mind.
    Most fifteen-year-olds would be warm in their beds on a cold October night. The heating had clicked off long ago. It was after two. I startled at every noise. Just as I eventually began to doze, I was alerted to something being thrown to his window from our driveway. Leaping up to investigate, I saw them: the aforementioned associates, concealed in hoods. I strained to hear their conversation.
    "He's ignoring us.
    "Maybe he's not there."
    "I'm not having this."
    "But he owes me."
    "We could just press the doorbell."
    "He told me he'd have some."
    "Nah, he'll keep."
    Crouching under the window, I hoped they had not seen me peering. Why wouldn't they just give up and leave my fractured family in peace? I had not yet turned off the lantern outside the front door. Until he was in, I always left it switched on. It cast unwelcome shards of light, stabbing me through the venetian blind.
    Becoming Tom's mother had robbed me of the right to sleep. Sixteen years on, I was still alone, in the dead of night. A solitary figure: enveloped in darkness, longing to be allowed to rest like all the others.

The First Sleepless Night

(January 1994, aged 0.5 days)

"At least they can go back to sleep," I thought, bitterly, as I observed them all in the darkness around my illuminated bed. It was 1.45am. Tom wriggled on my bed, all flailing arms and legs. But at least he had stopped crying for now.

By 2.30, I was desperate to sleep. I had fed and changed him three times, cuddled him and tried laying him down, both in his cot and in bed with me. Tugging on my dressing gown, I lowered my bare feet onto the cold floor. I gathered him up again and lay his tiny, warm form upright against my shoulder. A little walk around was sure to settle him.

The ward was in darkness except for a dim lamp at the nurse's station and the fairy lights on the Christmas tree. I held him towards them, hoping for distraction. He quietened and fastened his stare upon the twinkling colours. The ward was in silence apart from the low buzz of conversation that occasionally passed between the nursing staff. A whiff of coffee and toast made my stomach inadvertently rumble. It must have been about thirty six hours since I had eaten, before my labour pains had begun.

"Shall we take him for a while?" offered one of nurses, standing up behind the high desk. "You need to rest. He should settle soon. Being born wears them out!"

"Well, it's certainly worn me out!" I padded to the side of the desk. "Are you sure?"

"Of course." She held her arms out for him. "Pass him here."

I gave him to her and scuttled back to bed. Quickly, flicking off the overhead lamp, I burrowed gratefully beneath the bedclothes and closed my eyes. Sleep washed over me as easily as tumbling water over stones. But, in what seemed like moments later, I was awoken to a snuffling sound in the cot beside me. As though a hedgehog was rooting for food.

Rubbing my eyes, I grappled on the bedside cabinet for my watch. 4.20. The nurse must have returned him as I slept. Lifting him from the cot, I tried to feed him again, hoping he would fall asleep as he took his milk. He didn't. After a while, I decided to take him back to the nurses. I climbed back into bed and tried to go to sleep. But his high-pitched wail was echoing through the ward. I sighed as I heard footsteps 'click-clacking' towards my bed.

"I thought I'd better bring him back before he wakes everybody! He just wants his mummy."

Taking him from her, I scanned the darkened room. The moonlight was filtering in between the blinds. It cast wobbly shadows over the sleeping forms; five mothers and five babies. I fed him again. The silence of the night was only broken by the occasional snore or a momentary small cry. This would be answered with milk, swiftly resulting in a contented baby.

But not mine. If any of the other new mothers had glanced over at my bed, they would have peered through the thin curtain, pulled around, in a fruitless attempt to mask the wails of an un-pacified child.

They would have noticed me, a jostling silhouette, trying to cajole my baby into sleep. Envy was not in their eyes. It was in mine.

The Second and Third Sleepless Nights

"It is most unusual," stated the doctor as she visited on her rounds, later that morning. "New babies are normally exhausted after birth. They hardly wake in the first few days, apart from to be fed or changed. I'm sure he will settle down for you though." She briskly moved to the next bed.

Tom had finally fallen asleep at about 5.30 that morning. Minutes later, or so it felt, the breakfast trolley had begun to rattle around. Feeling nauseous from tiredness, I had managed a bit of toast and marmalade. Its tang lingered in my mouth as I nestled back onto the pillows.

I peeked into Tom's cot. Still he slept. He was now into his fourth hour of sleep since being born thirty eight hours before.

As I lay down amidst the warm ward, I was so worn out that I could hardly hear the chattering of the other mums to each other. The doorbell to the ward buzzed constantly. I knew it was happening but it was somewhat peripheral.

Peter's voice beside me made me jump.

"Come on sleepy, the doctor has come to see you both." He peered into the cot. "Hello little man."

"What, again?" I hauled myself up from the pillow. "The doctor's already checked him."

"You're coming home son!" He scooped Tom up. "He needs a final once over, that's all."

Peter had brought Tom's car seat, all-in-one coat and his bobble hat. Once we had been checked and discharged, a nurse accompanied us to the hospital foyer to help us into the taxi. My eyes ached, hit by the sudden glaze, as I exchanged the artificial light for winter sunshine. It was a beautiful day, perfect to take our baby home.

The peace and warmth would enable Tom to settle better. I eagerly anticipated being back in my own bed with Peter to lend a hand during the night feeds. But I was to be disappointed. Peter slumbered nonchalantly through Tom's nocturnal noise ensuring even less sleep was afforded to me than had been in hospital. I fed him until sore and rocked him until I wept. I felt exasperated and powerless and was desperate to close my eyes and rest.

At some point I must have fallen asleep because abruptly, I awoke to find the room in quiet stillness. Jumping up, I lunged towards Tom's sleeping basket. It was empty. I ran into the kitchen and spotted a note by the kettle.

"Taken Tom to meet my mum. Get some rest."

Of course he meant well. But fury speared me. We should have *both* taken Tom to meet his grandma. Looking around our home, it seemed rest would be the last thing I could get. The place was a tip. Every available surface was covered in baby paraphernalia. Laundry and the dishes needed attending to. Peter must have done nothing before heading out with Tom. I sobbed as I clattered around. The cleaner and tidier my flat became; the more my mood darkened. I could not shake it.

It continued all day. Peter ran me a bath later that evening. I wallowed in it, weeping as I listened to the bubbles in the foam popping. My tears were as warm as the bath water.

"I'm going to buy milk powder so I can feed him tonight. You're going to get a proper night's sleep." His voice suddenly cut into my thoughts from the bathroom door.

It made me feel like a failure to be depriving Tom of breast milk. This self-reproach threatened to overpower me. However he seemed to like the formula and guzzled greedily from the bottle, gazing wide-eyed at Peter as he suckled. I tunnelled beneath the bedclothes, appreciative that he was having a turn at being kept awake.

By ten past four, the formula had run out. There were no more bottles sterilised. Peter nudged me as Tom squawked from his basket.

"You'll have to sort him Sarah. I've had enough." He turned and faced the other way. "I need some sleep."

Bleary eyed, I reluctantly retrieved him. There was no more sleep for me that night.

As the weeks limped over each other, we became different people. We no longer laughed. We barely conversed. We snapped. We fought. We compared. We blamed.

He slept. I didn't. He worked. I coped. The gulf widened and by the time Tom was five months old, reality had to be confronted. Head on.

"I need a break from you." I bawled at him, overwhelmed by fatigue and responsibility. "I can't stand you around me at the moment."

"I'll stay at my mum's for a couple of weeks." After thundering from the room, he slammed around for a while as he packed his possessions.

His leaving came too easily. I sensed a whiff of relief. Respite from his newly acquired middle-aged lifestyle. Me, I just had to get on with it.

The 182nd Sleepless Night

(August 1994, aged 8 months)

After Peter's departure, Tom 'slept' in bed with me. Six, seven or eight times a night, he would wake, for twenty to thirty minute periods. Then, he would doze for about twenty minutes before stirring again. I don't know why he kept waking. His nappy did not need changing and milk would be rejected. It was necessary to accept this situation and resign myself to this way of life. In hindsight, I do not know how I kept functioning.

The weather had improved so the windows were often ajar. His incessant crying must have disturbed the neighbours. If this was the case, no one ever protested. They may have felt sorry for me. Or wondered what I was doing wrong.

Had they had peered through their windows, they would have witnessed us in the street on many a night. As early dawn broke, Tom would bawl from his buggy, as I paced up and down the pavement, trying to lull him to sleep using the wheeled motion.

I hope nobody noticed me on one particular occasion. My mood was as black as the cortex of the night. I howled outwardly in frustration. Neighbours may have questioned why I was alone.

Has she left her baby on his own? I had been forced to. I had come close to hurting him. My rage had been so powerful that I had been able to taste it. It had tingled in my nose with the ferocity of a nose bleed. A white madness had engulfed me before I had fled from the flat, innately aware that if I did not get away from him, I might have hurled him against the wall.

"Will you shut up?" I had shoved him a little too roughly into his cot. In complete anguish, I then circled the street. The regret consumed me. *I had nearly hurt my baby!* I had allowed anger to devour my exhaustion and the adrenaline had cascaded through my veins.

After I had calmed enough to return to him, he had cried himself out. So had I. Gently drawing him towards me, I kissed the top of his head.

"I'm sorry baby. Please forgive me. I could never hurt you. Ever." Rocking him in the darkness, I wept into his hair, breathing his powdery, pure scent. There was no way that could ever happen again. I *had* to come to terms with my new existence.

The next day was spent making a remorseful fuss of him; playing and singing with him more than usual.

Despite the angst, I adored Tom. My world revolved around him. Every spare penny was spent on new toys and lovely outfits. He was my blue-eyed, white- haired everything.

SURELY MOTHERHOOD SHOULDN'T BE THIS HARD??

An Active Child

Like an Olympic swimmer, Tom mastered the art of the crawl with equal speed and finesse and could not, even momentarily, be left unattended. Everything had to be shifted. Everything! Ornaments, photographs, magazines, the cat's food dish and all that could be spilt. Have you ever had to do a risk assessment for your entire home and everything in it? Anything within his grasp was at risk. It was as though he organised his next onslaught in his mind as I changed his nappy.

Every day would be like a scene from 'The Great Escape.' Held prisoner in my arms, I became used to the ferocious wriggling and determined attempts to break free – this was his usual response to being detained. When captured, he would wriggle ferociously and then as soon as he was free, would escape across the room at a breathtaking pace towards anything inadvertently left out that might attract his eye. On his hands and knees, he would hurtle towards a coveted item that he could wrench apart, pour or throw. Even the cat, once curious at him, kept a safe distance.

He was clearly mobile at ten months; the health visitor seemed amazed.

"He's advanced for his age." She watched in astonishment as he waddled towards her. "I can't believe he's walking already!" *'Welcome to my world!'* I desperately wanted to reply. Instead, I breathed in deeply and fixed my expression: a strange combination of acceptance and exhaustion.

"Oh yes! I've got my hands full now!" I shuffled around the room, collecting discarded items as we talked.

"How's he sleeping?" She yanked her handbag away from Tom. "Dare I ask?"

"Still badly, but I'm used to it." I slung toys into his toy box and wondered if she detected the resignation in my voice.

"Has he slept through the night yet?" She tugged a form and a pen from her bag. I chuckled politely before disappearing into the kitchen to pour the coffee.

"I think the longest he's slept is for an hour!" I called out.

"It must be difficult for you."

No of course not! He's a breeze! What makes you think that having a child who sleeps for an hour a night is difficult? Inside the sarcasm bubbled away but I remained my jovial self, leaving the veil that cloaked the reality of my feelings firmly in place.

"I'm used to it now!" I no longer questioned it. It was my normality. I came back in with our drinks; she placed hers on the low table beside her.

"Will it be ok there?"

"No! Quick! Grab it!" She rescued it just in time as Tom took full swing.

This was one of his favourite games. He loved to swipe at cups and glasses and would approach them at remarkable speed. Before I had any chance of preventing him, he would have reached his target normally. Anything left within his grasp would be smashed. Digging up plants and ripping into books were also pursuits he particularly enjoyed.

Being confined in the bath was something he detested though. He would try to clamber out, or would thrash about in the water with a intensity that resembled a beached fish. Inevitably, I and the bathroom floor would be saturated. Therefore baths were a brief affair.

Restraint was necessary for all 'simple' tasks such as nappy changing, dressing and the putting on of shoes. Tom was strong and would squirm to be free. To watch me trying to strap him into his pushchair could be likened to a policeman trying to handcuff a newly captured criminal!

It was a challenging situation, but one I had to resign myself to. Surely this was how it must be for all new mums.

If I tried to visit people with Tom, excuses were politely made. Like *'we're just on our way out'* or *'I'm not well'* or *'we're expecting visitors in ten minutes.'* That kind of thing.

One friend was not so gracious. She had two boisterous little girls and Tom would be wild with anticipation whenever he encountered them. They fed off each others enthusiasm yet would have fared better if given space to rampage around in, rather than the confines of a cluttered living room.

One day, I visited and my friend invited me in.

"Mark's decided he must stay strapped in his buggy." She avoided eye contact with me as she informed me of her partner's wishes, just as I bent down to release Tom. "Every time he comes he breaks things or pours something. Or both. Perhaps it's better if we visit you in future."

Making my excuses, I left, blinkered with tears, before trudging round to another friend's house to repeat the conversation. She was sympathetic. But her partner wasn't.

"I don't blame him for saying that." I heard him mutter as Tom threw his bottle of juice at one of their framed pictures, smashing it. As I left, I decided not to visit in future if her partner's car was outside.

It was becoming like that everywhere. I was increasingly isolated. People insisted on visiting me rather than risking the damage that my son might inflict. At least in my own home, it was *my* stuff getting smashed. Not that I had much left!

It was fruitless attempting a shopping trip too; or meeting a friend, for a cup of tea in a café; or queuing in the post office. Every activity would be blighted by Tom's screams for attention. Arching his back in temper, he would repeatedly hurl his head against the back of his buggy. God only knows how he did not injure himself. People would gape at us and mutter about his behaviour which made me feel like even more of an outcast.

Especially one Sunday when we attended church. We didn't go often as it was too much of an ordeal. However, there were some Sundays when I felt compelled to go. I loved the peace and stillness. The scent of incense would wash over me as soon as I entered. It was a relief to sit in the quiet. If only Tom would have permitted this!

We lingered at the back, so as not to interrupt the service. I was armed with juice, biscuits and a couple of noiseless toys. Five minutes into the service, the commotion he was causing forced me to drag him outside. My teeth clattered in the icy air as I attempted to calm him down. Our coats, of course, were inside.

Whilst a hymn was being sung, we ventured back in. As soon as it was over, Tom fired up again. He squawked an excruciatingly loud 'NO!!' and writhed in anger, as I tried to keep a hold on his squirming little body. My face burned and I knew I had to get us out of there. Every eye was on me, in silent condemnation.

Just as I was gathering our things together, an elderly woman barged over, coming so close to us that her perfume penetrated the incense.

"What do you think you're doing? I've come here to listen to the service, not the likes of that!" Her finger jabbed sharply towards me. She glared at Tom as though he was diseased. It was a reaction I had to get used to, quickly. The pain in the top of my chest felt as though I had swallowed a sob and it had gone down the wrong way.

"What is it Jesus said?" remarked another woman, jumping to my defence. "*Suffer the little children who come unto me.* "Ignore her," she implored. "You're as welcome here as she is,"

But there was no way. The damage was done. It was years before I ventured back into a church.

Baby's First Christmas

"Look at our gorgeous tree!" Balancing Tom's weight on my hip, I ambled over to where it proudly presided. For several seconds, he stared at the lights, their assorted colours reflecting onto the perfection of his face. I was transported back in time, to the nurses' station where he had, as a newborn, gazed at the tree there. He swung his arm at one of the baubles.

"No Tom!" I caught hold of his arm. "Don't spoil the tree!" He began to wriggle in order to get me to lower him to the floor.

"I'll get you a drink," I announced, finally putting him down. He had to get used to the tree, and would probably tug at its adornments but seriously, what damage could he do?

If you slowly count to twenty now, you will get an idea of the length of my absence from the room. As I made the short journey back from the kitchen to the living room, there was a crash, not a loud one but a 'tinselly' one.

"Tom!" I raced back into the room. "No!"

He stepped back from the tree, still aglow on the floor and appeared to be admiring his handiwork.

"That's naughty!" He giggled as I tapped his hand. Leading him to his room, I plonked him in his cot, ignoring his wails as I put the tree back together.

On releasing him, I shouted "no!" whenever he approached it and tapped his hand when he was about to make a grab for one of its ornaments. As I prepared his tea, he got another opportunity. Once again, the tree sprawled forlornly upon the carpet. Protecting it grew tiresome and I was glad when 'bedtime' was approaching.

This night, like every night, after his tea, I bathed him, and tried to settle him in his room with a bottle. As I sang, he would whinge, all too aware of the inevitable. Then I would have to 'peel' him from me. His fingers would grip onto my clothing, similar to an abandoned chimpanzee, to prevent me from laying him down. I had to be firm.

Back in the living room, I would crank up the TV's volume, in an effort to drown out his screaming. But he would repeatedly throw his head against the bars of his cot. This was impossible to ignore so I would give in and retrieve him. This process would last throughout the evening, into the early hours and was repeated nightly.

His bedroom was gradually ruined as he enjoyed ripping the wallpaper within reach around his cot. Both of his musical cot mobiles had been pulled down along with the toys I had secured to the bars.

Christmas Eve was not as I would have envisaged. Tom's first Christmas. My tree stood bedraggled and unlit, worn out from being mercilessly thrown. Not as worn out as me though. I was twenty one years-old, yet felt about seventy one. Other girls would be out partying tonight. Unlike me: huddled on the sofa, surrounded by darkness, with just a glass of wine for company.

The only light wavered in the corner of the room, from the TV. Closing my eyes and scrunching them tightly did not eliminate the screaming and endless banging coming from the little bedroom. But I had to ignore it. Enough was enough.

It was a relief to welcome the arrival of the new year; and with it, Tom's first birthday. At around this time, he managed to 'break out' of his cot. I could not believe it when he came tearing into the living room one night, waving his bottle.

"Bot-bot!" I re-filled it with orange juice and hauled him back to bed, where I was astonished to find that he had snapped two of the bars on his cot. After that, there was no hope of confining him in his room at bedtime.

"Bot-bot!" he would bawl as he raced out of his room up to eight times every night. I would present him with orange juice and return him to his room. His thirst started to concern me. It was insatiable and his nappies were saturated!

Soon, I discarded his cot for a bed. I slept on a knife's edge, poised the whole time for disturbance. People commented on my sunken face and dark eyes, caused by a year of no sleep. I wondered if it was ever going to end.

One February morning, I awoke with a start and glanced at the clock. 7. 45 am. He had not woken since midnight! I shot across the hallway of our flat into his room and shook him. He remained in stillness.

For a moment I thought he was dead.

"Tom!" I screeched. Panic shrouded me as I shook him again. He sprang up like a jack-in-a box. "Bot-bot! He thrust the bottle at me. I hugged him in relief!

Happily, two or three times each week, he began to sleep through the main part of the night and was starting to allow me four to five hours of uninterrupted sleep. Rather than wake in a blind panic, I felt utter gratitude. However, I knew I would never take sleep for granted again.

Does orange juice cause hyperactivity?

Symptoms of Hyperactivity

IN INFANCY

- Crying screaming, restless, needs little sleep.
- Colic. Difficult to feed, whether breast or bottle.
- Cannot be pacified or cuddled... spurns affection.
- Excessive dribbling... may be VERY THIRSTY.
- Head banging, cot rocking, fits and tantrums.

OLDER CHILDREN (in addition to symptoms in infancy)

- Clumsy, impulsive.., accident prone.
- Erratic disruptive behaviour.
- Compulsive 'touching'. Constant motion.
- Disturbs other children. May be aggressive.
- Lacks concentration and may be withdrawn.
- Normal or high I.Q. but fails at school.
- Poor appetite. Poor hand and eye co-ordination.
- Uncooperative, defiant and disobedient.
- Self abusive (pulling hair/picking skin etc.).
- Continued problems with sleep.

There are, of course, degrees of the problem, and not every child will have all the symptoms described here. More boys than girls are hyperactive. Figures show a ratio of 3:1 (high percentage of blonde blue eyed boys).

(Source: Hyperactive Children's Support Group)

He Should Be Muzzled!

May 1995 (1 year, 5 months)

As the days lengthened, I began to feel more positive. I coerced myself out of the flat with Tom, even if it was just to the park so he could let off steam. Here I would sometimes bump into a friend and we could chat as Tom ran amok.

One friend, Cathy, was someone I met regularly. Her son, Jack, was six weeks older than Tom. He was a handful but not in the same league! I noticed one difference the first time I invited them for tea. The boys had spaghetti and sausages. Jack sat still at the table and fed himself with a spoon, albeit messily. But he concentrated.

Tom, however, had to be fastened into his highchair. His food was served in a bowl with a 'suction plate,' to stick it to his highchair tray. Within three seconds of receiving his meal, it lay splashed around the feet of the highchair on the plastic sheeting I had begun to use to protect the carpet. I scooped it up and tried again. To no avail.

I spooned it back into the bowl and tried to feed it to him myself. He screamed, arched his back in temper and spat out any food that did make it into his mouth.

"Is he always like this?" Cathy looked astonished as she wiped Jack's mouth.

"I'm afraid so." I let a jagged breath out. "I don't even try to eat my meal with him anymore!"

"Perhaps he's just not hungry," she suggested, frowning at him.

"He must be!" I held the spoon again against his clamped mouth. "He's not eaten for hours. I'd hoped he might improve with Jack setting such a good example."

"Maybe that's why he's doing it?" She lifted Jack out of the chair and clasped him towards her. "Maybe he's showing off!"

"No, he's like this every single mealtime!" I put the bowl aside, finally admitting defeat.

"Poor you!" She looked at me sympathetically. "Maybe you should just take the food away when he launches his bowl. He'll soon learn that he goes hungry when he does that!

"I've tried that already. He doesn't seem to learn anything, no matter what I do."

"Then keep trying. After a couple of days he'll get the message."

"I know you're only trying to help Cathy but honestly, I know what I'm doing." *Did I?*

Because our sons were similar in age, we often got together. We would feed the ducks or go to a soft indoor play area. Early one morning, Cathy phoned me with a suggestion:

"How about we take the bus to the coast?"

I glanced out of the window. "Well it's certainly sunny enough for it."

"I'll meet you at the bus stop in an hour."

My mood was as cheerier than the day outside as I bundled together everything we would need. It would be wonderful to get some sea air! As I bustled around the flat, Tom sprawled before the TV, nibbling at his toast.

"No!" I admonished as I re-entered the room; to discover he was stuffing it into the video recorder.

Every ounce of my strength was required to strap him into his buggy. But eventually, we were organised. Cathy and Jack were waiting at the bus stop.

Throughout the first bus ride, Tom squirmed on my knee, yearning for escape. Cathy twisted herself so that her upper half and Jack were almost facing into the aisle between the seats in what, I suppose, was an attempt to distance herself from us as all the other passengers who were staring at Tom in distaste. I prayed he would sleep on the longer trip we were to embark on. It was to take ninety minutes!

Cathy and I perched on the second bus with our sons on our laps. Ten minutes into the journey, Tom had had enough and was on a mission to be free which was obviously not possible. His body was tense with rage and I had to shield my face from injury as he repeatedly flung his head backwards. Then he leant forwards and yanked the hair of a passenger in front.

"I'm sorry!" I gasped. "Are you alright?"

She raked some of the hair that he had torn from her scalp and held it in front of me.

"That," she snarled "is disgusting! You ought to get him sorted out!" She yanked her bag from the overhead rack before making towards the steps to shift to an upstairs seat.

Tom's behaviour was having a terrible effect on Jack, who was beginning to wriggle and grimace in a similar way to him. At one point they were causing such a commotion that the bus driver screeched the bus to a halt.

"You're going to have to control those kids!" Twisting around, he surveyed us in revulsion. "I can't concentrate! What's bloody wrong with em both? Have you given em drugs or something?"

"Hear, hear!" agreed a couple sat behind us. I glanced at Cathy. Clearly unfamiliar to being shamed in this way, she concealed her crimson face behind Jack's head.

"I'll move to the seat in front with him I think," she muttered, sliding towards it without looking at me. For the rest of the journey, she did not speak. I doubt I'd have been able to hear her above the din Tom kept making anyway.

Had I been on a local bus, I would have got off and waited for the next one. The day seemed to be ruined before it had begun. Finally we reached our destination. I had never felt so grateful.

"He should be muzzled." A man snapped, as we descended.

"You can say that again." An elderly woman surveyed me coldly, shaking her head. "I hope we're on a different bus to you when we go home!"

"Do you really have to be so nasty?" Tears swam into my eyes. "Haven't you had kids of your own?"

"Not like that one!"

"Have you ever heard of parenting classes?" A younger woman shouted after me.

Turning abruptly, I had barely opened my mouth in response when Cathy grabbed my arm.

"Just ignore her! I've had enough embarrassment for one day!"

The prospect of the return journey blighted our day out. Cathy was cooler towards me and barely spoke to Tom. She even took herself off with Jack's buggy for an hour, her reasoning being that Jack was unable to take his afternoon nap around Tom.

Thankfully, our return home was less problematic. Jack slumbered for most of it in his mother's arms. Again, Cathy sat in a different seat. Any other passengers would have assumed we were strangers rather than two friends having the day out with our children.

I was surprised that Tom did not nod off, given his day of relentless activity in the sea air. However he was more manageable than earlier that day, tantrumming only a handful of times, as opposed to constantly. Mercifully, the bus was only half-full, allowing people to move away from us if they wished.

First Bid For Freedom

Tom seemed weary as I bathed him that evening. Not in his usual frenzied mood. I read him a story as he guzzled milk from his bottle, then I kissed him before drawing his curtains. The fading sunlight seeped into their edges like an eclipsed moon.

Being a muggy evening, I opened his window slightly then clicked his door shut behind me. Momentarily, he grizzled but he did not pursue me out of the room. Within twenty minutes, all was peaceful. Tucking my feet under me, I curled up gratefully in front of the TV, wondering whether to celebrate my success at getting him to sleep with a cheeky glass of wine or bar of chocolate. I glanced happily at an untouched magazine that I had not had a moment to enjoy. Until tonight.

Minutes later, on the edge of my vision, I noticed a woman hauling a child across the grassed area that our flat overlooked. My heart began hammering against my rib cage as I realised it was Tom. Time seemed to slow as I scrambled out of my chair and began fumbling beyond the red mist that had descended for my door keys. *How on earth had this woman managed to abduct my son?*

I pelted to the door, and darted across the grass towards her.

"Stop! Stop!" My shrieks sounded as though they belonged to someone else.

"Is he yours?" she screeched as he tugged and squirmed for escape.

"Yes. What ……." I yanked him from her by the arm, scarcely able to breathe.

"You stupid woman! Can't you look after your own child? I've just stopped him being killed."

"I thought he was asleep!" My face was smouldering as I clutched him towards me. "Honestly, I only tucked him into bed ten minutes ago." I sounded pathetic. "He must have climbed through his window."

"Well thanks a lot anyway!" She began striding away, shaking her head. "I've just missed my bus because of you."

"I'm so sorry!" Tear flamed my eyes. Tears of humiliation or grief, I was not sure.

"Well you can fish your own kid off the road next time." She shouted back over her shoulder. "You're a disgrace!"

Open mouthed, I stared after her. It was horrendous being yelled at, being blamed. Mostly I was ashamed and realised how I must have appeared. *How could I have argued?*

Tom, pyjama-clad, was a picture of innocence. It was a battle to keep a grip of him as I carted him back to the flat; he was battling to get free again.

He *had* climbed out of his bedroom window. It was an absolute mercy that we lived in the ground floor flat of the high rise block. He must have clambered from his bed, onto his windowsill and descended the five feet onto the grass outside. It was amazing! *How on earth could an eighteen-month-old child safely drop five feet? Thank God that woman had seen him! The alternatives did not bear contemplating!* Nestled within my relief was guilt that I had not pre-empted this possibility. After that, I never left his window ajar again.

Good Morning!

September 1995 (1 year, 9 months)

Mornings were incredibly tough. Especially if I had not been allowed much sleep during the night. Usually, within a short while of waking, Tom would pelt into my room and demand the replenishment of his 'bot-bot.' Then he began to establish a new routine.

The first time it occurred, I had lain, semi conscious, hearing a scuffling in the kitchen. I was not awake enough to act upon it. But after an almighty crash, I scurried in to investigate. Flinging open the door, the sight before me made me gasp.

Covered in cat food and smeared in margarine, Tom sprawled, cross-legged, in a heap of tipped-out Persil. The kitchen looked as though it had been burgled. In a sense, I suppose, it had. All six yogurts had been devoured and the cheese block gnawed at. Most of the fridge's contents lay strewn across the floor. A cup of tea was not an option as the carton of milk had been emptied everywhere.

This became a regular occurrence, so within days, I fitted fridge and cupboard locks, also ensuring everything in the kitchen was out of Tom's reach.

The morning after the locks had been installed; another jolt awaited me upon awakening.

I emerged from my room, stunned to note that he was still in his room.

"Tom, breakfast time." I opened his door. Then I discovered what he had done "You naughty, dirty little boy!"

The contents of his nappy had been smeared everywhere. It adorned his bed, walls, the floor and himself. The overpowering stink made me gag. Closing the door for a moment gave me the space to take a few gulps of air and compose myself.

Then, when I reopened the door, with my jumper over my face, I was primed for the stench that whacked me like a sledgehammer!

Pinning him down, I scraped the worst from him with baby wipes as I waited for the bath to fill. Unfortunately, this little 'game' also grew habitual. It was as though he was trying to punish me.

"Perhaps he's trying to tell you he's ready to be potty trained," suggested the health visitor, wrapping her fingers around her mug of tea. By now, she had learned to keep hold of it! Although when I recounted his other escapades, particularly his tendency to escape, she was alarmed!

"You must make sure you keep all the doors and windows locked." Her gaze flicked around the room as she spoke.

"I do." I scooped Tom up and dumped him on my knee. I had sensed he was about to investigate the contents of the health visitor's handbag by how he was appraising it. "But then he bangs his head when he can't have his own way."

"Now that is worrying." Placing her cup beside her, she extracted a notebook from her bag. "How often is he doing that?"

"Every day really." I lowered Tom back to the floor. Clearly he did not want to sit on my knee. "Sometimes he bangs on his wall, sometimes it's against the floor or if we are out, he throws his head back against the buggy. It's particularly bad at bed time though."

We both surveyed Tom who had hurtled over to his toy box and was flinging his toys onto the floor with great gusto.

"How would you react if I was to suggest putting in a referral to the 0-19 Team?"

I chewed my bottom lip and nervously raised my eyes to hers. "What does that mean?"

"They're specialists with problem behaviour. Hopefully they'll be able to give you some advice." She was scribbling onto her notepad as she chatted to me.

"I'm not sure." I paused, lost in thought for a moment. "I'm doing all I can with him." I glanced around at my cluttered and unkempt living room, which smelt of old milk and baby wipes. "I tell him off. I watch him like a hawk." My voice faded. "I'm scared they'll blame me."

"Of course they won't." Reaching over, she rested her hand on my arm. "You're doing a wonderful job. But you do need support."

"I know." I felt drained. I reluctantly agreed she could refer him. There was certainly nothing else on offer.

Second Bid for Freedom

Tom was quietly playing in his room. Being that it was the middle of the day and he had seemed a little subdued after lunch, I had hoped he might take a little afternoon nap which would enable me to get a few jobs done. As I folded the laundry into a pile, I glimpsed absently out of the window, suddenly dropping it all when I spotted a workman dragging Tom from the road.

This time, I knew abduction was not a possibility, he must have undone the catch on his window himself. I tore across the grass, berating myself for another furious onslaught.

"I'm sorry!" I tried to get in before he could unleash the condemnation that was evident in his expression. "He's done this before! I'm going to nail his window down!" I struggled to get my words out between my gasps for air."

"You want reporting, you do. Look at the size of him! Thank God I saw him when I did!"

"I know how it must look. I'm really sorry!"

"You will be when he gets run over. You ought to be ashamed of yourself!"

This time I could not hold back the tears as I trudged away, wrestling to hang onto my wriggling child. There was no point trying to convince this man of anything. He shared a common opinion. I was useless, useless, useless!

The tears rolled down my cheeks and the more I tried to quell them, the faster they spilt.

The 0-19 Team

"What triggers him to bang his head?" The man peered over his spectacles as Tom tipped out the entire toy box with a crash.

"Usually when he's upset." Tom sifted through the toys, searching for one which appealed to him.

"What sort of things is he upset by?" The man crossed his legs, which were clad in trousers boasting a pristine crease down the centre, socks sporting a diamond pattern and the shiniest shoes I had ever seen.

I shuffled awkwardly in my chair. "Mealtimes, bedtime, bath time; being made to sit in his buggy." Tom was becoming restless as he lolled among the discarded toys. I resisted the urge to attend to him. "Anything."

"Do you tell him off?" As he posed the question, he ducked just in time to allow a carefully aimed toy to skim the top of his receding head. His expectant expression conveyed that he expected me to do something about this.

"Of course I tell him off – it's all I ever seem to do." I leaned over to where Tom sat, beaming mischievously at a pair of scissors he had discovered in the toy box. I confiscated them and thrust them at the man.

"Do you smack him?" He gently placed the scissors in a drawer.

"I sometimes shout or smack his hand." I expected the man to approve but he stared at me with distaste.

"We don't condone smacking, you know." I tried to see what he was scribbling on his clipboard but he protectively raised it towards his chest.

"I meant *tap* his hand." Perhaps in adding that he would alter *shocking mother* to *not-so-bad mother!*

"He is lively," he remarked, watching Tom who was amusing himself by grabbing and hurling items from the man's desk. "No, please don't do that," the man implored politely, as he bent to retrieve a hole punch from his grasp. Normally I would have intervened but I wanted him to glimpse Tom in full throttle.

"I'm worried there's something wrong," I asserted as the man gave up and allowed Tom to retain the hole punch. "He's constantly on the go. He sleeps terribly and destroys whatever he can get his hands on."

"I see. And he's not even two yet?" The man looked irked as a million tiny white circles suddenly littered his immaculate green carpet.

"No." I outstretched my hand to Tom for the hole punch.

"Have you thought about trying a parenting course?" The man fished around in his briefcase.

I chewed my lip in an attempt to quell the expletive that was threatening to be spoken. This was an utter waste of time. The man was useless. I concluded the appointment, adamant that I would sort him out myself.

I would be stricter and enforce a tighter routine. Everything would be kept out of his way and more locks would be fitted. Whatever it took to manage him better would be implemented. But there were always going to be occasions when I would need to relax my vigilance.

When we got home, I poured Tom a drink and switched on the TV. Normally I would have put on a video tape on to amuse him. Unfortunately, just days before, the machine had grown exhausted of being stuffed with food and toys. It was ready to join the growing list of Tom's breakages.

"Just sit there sweetheart. Mummy's nipping to the loo. Won't be a moment."

Within seconds, there was a deafening bang. Sprinting back into the room, I saw that Tom had lodged himself behind the cabinet and shoved the TV onto the floor. It smoked and sparked as though it was a maddened volcano.

I flew towards Tom, grabbed him and raced with him over to the door. The TV made a peculiar popping noise before it died.

"Great. Thanks very much." I inhaled the scent of the smoking TV. Listening to the radio was not an option either as Tom had previously snapped the aerial. He always seemed to target items that would be expensive to replace. It was soul destroying.

Extra Parent 1 (A reluctant Stepfather)

Martin

Parking my car, I advanced towards the door of her flat. A child's shrieks amplified with every step.

"Hello stranger!" Sarah flung the door open. With wild hair and an even wilder child under her arm, she looked at me. He was battling to get free. After a moment, she released him and he bolted off. She wore a floor-length skirt with what appeared to be a nightie over it.

"I'm sorry," she reddened, glancing down at herself as she dragged her fingers through her hair. "I haven't had chance to get dressed properly yet!"

"Don't worry." I twisted my car key within my fingers. "I should've rung first."

"Come in." The door opened a little wider. "I'll put the kettle on."

I followed her inside. Her little boy was racing in a zigzag fashion from one wall of the room to the other and back again. He had clearly been on the rampage. Curtains were half hung and cups were overturned. Strewn toys and clothes carpeted the floor. God knows what was smeared on a window and a picture had been smashed. It was as though a tornado had ripped through the room, damaging everything in its path. But this tornado was still escalating.

"Enough!" Sarah screeched at him, looking worn out and incredibly stressed.

"You make some tea." I strode towards him. "I'll keep an eye on him." I promised.

As she left the room, I caught him in mid flight and bent down. "Hello." As I attempted to engage his gaze, the marble-like appearance of his eyes struck me. His pupils were so dilated; it was difficult to distinguish his eye colour. My phone fell from my top pocket. Tom immediately seized it.

"No. No Tom!" Backing away with my phone, he had an evil sneer on his lips. "Give it to me," I coaxed, moving towards him.

Raising his arm, he launched it at the wall. Bolting towards it, I managed to retrieve it before he did. Luckily, it seemed unscathed.

"You've got your hands full!" My expression must have been loaded with sympathy for Sarah, who had returned to the living room bearing two mugs of tea. Tom was now vaulting from the window sill onto the sofa."

"I know." She passed me a mug before sinking down onto a chair.

"Perhaps I could call round one evening when he's in bed?" I suggested, as I sipped my tea. "Then we can have a proper catch up." Then as an afterthought, I added, "I'll bring wine." She looked as though she could do with some!

"Yes." I was relieved she did not balk at my offer. "That'd be lovely. Only be warned," she glared at her son, "it's not always simple to get Tom to bed."

I arranged to return at the weekend. As I unlocked my car, I shook my head in disbelief, unable to believe what Sarah was coping with. *What a nightmare of a child!* I was one hundred per cent convinced that there was something not right with him.

On Friday, I returned to Sarah's. As I approached, it was heartening to notice that Tom's window was curtained and no wailing was audible.

"Ssshh!" she raised a finger to her lips upon answering the door. "He's asleep."

I tiptoed through the hallway and she clicked the living room door behind me.

"I'll get some glasses," she announced, spotting the wine I was clutching. Her living room was in much better shape than it had been before. As I poised to perch on the sofa, there were several blobs of what appeared to be nail varnish. Gingerly, I lowered myself next to it.

"Oh, I stupidly left a bottle of nail varnish out. It was so upsetting; the sofa was new. I've not even finished paying for it yet!"

A cracked window caught my attention. "Don't tell me he's done that as well!"

"I'm afraid so!" She followed my gaze. "He chucked his bottle at it."

I shook my head. "How old is he now?"

"He'll be two in six weeks!" She passed me a corkscrew and I began uncorking the wine.

Tom must have sensed he was being discussed, for at that moment, he burst in through the door.

"Bot-bot!" The bottle he launched nearly struck his mother. Retrieving it, she headed to the kitchen.

I waited for about ten minutes, listening to his fierce screams. Sarah seemed to be trying to settle him back to bed. Finally, she re-emerged with him balanced on one hip.

"It's no good. He's wide awake!" She gestured towards the glass I clutched. "Just make sure you keep that in your hand!"

I left soon after. It was apparent that Tom was not going to back down. I liked Sarah but could not help feeling more than a bit repelled by her son.

Third Bid for Freedom

I was taking no chances with Tom's safety after his previous break-outs and had therefore nailed down his bedroom window. Of course, he discovered an alternative escape: the balcony, which our external living room door opened onto. Never would I have imagined he could possibly climb over the railings, let alone negotiate the six foot drop at the other side. Visiting friends looked dubious when I showed them the height from which he had jumped or lowered himself.

One evening, I began washing the dishes whilst leaving Tom surrounded by the contents of his upturned toy box. Whether he would actually play with them or just launch them over the balcony was debateable but at least he was quiet for now. Inhaling the floral scent of washing up liquid, I gazed absently through the window. My attention was suddenly diverted to the din of yelling and car horns. Craning my neck, I tried to see what was going on, suspecting that there must have been an accident.

An all-too-familiar blonde head became visible amongst several stationary vehicles. Even though I knew it was him, I still glanced into the living room in case I was mistaken and he was innocently playing with his toys. I could barely catch my breath as I hurtled out of the flat towards the commotion.

It was as though time slowed as I tried to get to him, terrified he'd been hurt. Within moments, I joined him in the centre of the road, yanking him from his feet into my arms. Angry rants from the occupants of surrounding cars echoed all around me. Even though I longed to defend myself I knew it would be futile. He was safe – that was the main thing. I gripped Tom tightly as the words of fury continued to be flung. Tom writhed in my arms like an abducted child, so much so, I am surprised no one challenged whether I was actually his mother.

Grimly, I placed one foot in front of the other, not daring to look back. Each jeer forced a fresh tear behind my eyes and I hoped to make it back into the flat before I let them slide down my face.

"You naughty, naughty boy!" I choked. He continued to wriggle.

In retrospect, I can understand the opinions of the onlookers; what an incompetent, irresponsible parent I must have seemed!

Fresh air within our home became a luxury I was forced to forsake. Any opportunity such as a door left ajar or a slightly open window obviously would prove too much for Tom to resist.

Aaarrghhh!

Extra Parent 2 – Elizabeth (surplus, saviour stepmother)

January 1996 (2 years)

I held a tea-party for Tom on his second birthday. One of his friends brought along an electronic Buzz Lightyear he had received at Christmas. When he wasn't allowed to keep it, Tom jealously wrench its arm out of its socket.

He bit two children, trapped the finger of another and one little girl lost a fistful of hair to him. Another of my living room windows met its demise when Tom hurled his new truck at it, then he narrowly escaped scorching himself when he made a sudden grab at his lit birthday cake. There was food splattered everywhere and I was relieved beyond words when the party ended.

The other mothers, all friends to me, must have sensed my stress and maintained a polite silence. One friend though, Tina, made a comment as she left that afternoon;

"Sarah, I'm not sure how you cope!" Wide-eyed, she surveyed at the debris that was left. "Is Tom's behaviour always this bad?"

"I'm hopeful he'll grow out of it," I held the door open for her. "I'm working on it anyway!" I joked half-heartedly, trying to conceal my shamed face behind my hair.

"I honestly don't think I could manage." She smugly clutched the hand of her well-behaved daughter. "I think you're brave for attempting a party!"

Later that day, Tom's dad turned up with his new girlfriend. It was a moment I had been dreading but was bound to happen at some point. She appeared younger than me. Having said that, I was so fatigued and stressed; I think anyone would have looked younger than me!

"Sarah, this is Elizabeth." Peter smirked nervously as he signalled towards her.

"Nice to meet you." I tried to smile through gritted teeth as I offered my hand. "Can I get you a drink?"

"No," Elizabeth seemed cautious and unsure of me. "Thanks, but we can't stay long."

"You'd be lucky to drink it anyway," laughed Peter as they breezed into the hallway. "Drinks don't last long around Tom!"

"So are you going to spend some time with him?" I asked Peter. "I'd prefer it if you could take him out." I held the door ajar so he could view Tom's handiwork. "I had a party and have a lot of cleaning to do."

"Oh my God," gasped Peter, surveying the wreckage. "Did you leave them all unattended?"

"Don't be stupid!" I began gathering food remains from under the table. "Anyway it wasn't all of them. It was mainly Tom!"

"Do you need a hand?" offered Elizabeth, ambling towards me. "I warmed to her, feeling perhaps we might have been friends if we had met in different circumstances.

"No, I'll be OK, but thanks." I scraped something dubious looking from the carpet.

"Would you like us to take him overnight," she continued, bending down beside him as he tore open the last of his presents. "I bet you could do with a break. We're staying at my parents tonight. I'm sure they'd love to meet him."

"Are you sure that's a good idea?" Peter looked reluctant. "You can see what he's capable of!"

"We can keep him in line, *surely*?" She began squashing wrapping paper into a carrier bag. I suddenly felt possessive.

"It's fine. Don't worry." Rising up from the floor, I wiped my hands on a paper napkin. "Just take him for a couple of hours so I can have a break."

We debated it for a while. Eventually I relented and packed an overnight bag for him. I felt devoid of all energy as I watched Peter wrestle with him, trying to get his coat on and fasten him into his pushchair.

There was now an option between a night out, where I could act youthful and carefree again. Or I could have an unwinding evening and a restful nights' sleep. However, I felt overcome by a deepening emptiness, not to mention, exhaustion.

I surveyed in sadness as Peter, Elizabeth and Tom strolled across the grass, away from my flat. To an unknown observer, they appeared like the little family unit that I, myself, had yearned for. I had to prevent myself bolting after them and demanding that Elizabeth hand my baby back. For a moment it was like she was stealing him from me. Tears flooded my eyes as she took over pushing the buggy. *She had my baby!* I felt bereft as I realised people would assume *she* was Tom's mummy.

<u>What sort of things might get you barred from a public house?</u>

1. Fighting?
2. Being in possession of illegal substances?
3. Being drunk and disorderly?
4. Vandalism?
5. Theft?
6. Underage drinking?
7. Climbing up onto a pool table, pulling down your trousers and urinating all over the pool table?

(If anyone has a tale of anyone getting barred from a pub younger than two-and-a-half, please let me know)

Marble up My Bum!

July 1996 (2 years, 7 months)

"Marble up my bum!" Tom sang from where he squatted on the carpet. "Marble up my bum!"

I peered at him. Surely not. A sensation of dread stole around me as I envisaged a trip to the accident and emergency department. Fortunately, I was spared the humiliation. After an hour of coaxing and bribery on my part, he pushed it back out into his potty.

His messing himself was relentless. I grew tempted to revert back to nappies. But he was actually potty trained and would go several days without 'an accident.' Whilst with his childminder, he never *once* soiled or wet himself.

Because of his frequent accidents, it was necessary to bath him twice daily, which was a nightmare. Although the tantrumming and clamouring to get out of the bath had subsided, he still poured water everywhere. But most problematic was that he had started to conduct his toileting whilst in the bath. I would sense from his face that he was 'straining.' I would whisk him out of the water and dump him on the toilet. Once, however, I momentarily left him, whilst I got shampoo from the cupboard. I re-entered the bathroom and was baffled to see him actually stood inside the toilet bowl. Meanwhile, particles of poo were floating around the bath!

Whenever I tried to keep a rein of Tom in a shop or at a bus stop he would bite me like an angry dog. But more worrying was his biting of other children. His childminder reported daily occurrences of it. And a horrible incident happened at my flat when Cathy had brought Jack to play.

As we chatted, the boys fought over a toy. Jack was bent forwards so Tom dropped his head onto Jack's back. I watched, rooted to the spot in horror as Tom bore his teeth into exposed skin above Jack's waistband. The skin whitened, stretched taut as the bite deepened. Cathy leapt to her feet and literally had to hook her fingers in between Tom's teeth and her son's skin to release his grip.

    Jack howled in agony. The injury took weeks to heal. Cathy barely looked at me as she left our flat with her sobbing little boy.

The Urinals

Martin

    Scene 1 *The Royal public house, tap room, babysitting Tom, watching match*

Man:	Is that your son with the blond hair?
Me:	(frantically looking around) Eh? No, he's my girlfriends. I'm just looking after him.
Man:	Well you're not doing a very good job. He's currently in the gents. I think he'll need a bath when you get him home.
Me:	(jumping to feet) Oh no, I was so engrossed in the football, I didn't realise how long he'd been in there!
Man:	(displaying expression of disgust) He's been climbing in the urinals and throwing air fresheners around.
Me:	(upon observation of a drenched and pungent Tom) Your mum's gonna go mad! Look at the state of you!

More about Mornings

Martin

August 1996 (aged 2 years, 8 months)

Respite was afforded for Sarah by virtue of three God-sends:

1. Her job
2. Tom's fortnightly overnight stay with his dad
3. His fortnightly babysitter

Of course we took full advantage of these Tom-free evenings and would try to have a night out. After all, Sarah was 23 and I, 26. Inevitably we would progress to a nightclub and return home a little the worse for wear at a ridiculous hour of the night. Looking back, this was madness when we had Tom to face the next day!

The flat would be wrecked; however the full horror of his destruction would not become apparent until we had sobered up the following morning.

Tom would then get up unheard. We must have been comatose not to be alerted as he rampaged through the flat. Balancing on his slide, he would then be able to reach the elevated kitchen door lock in order to empty the fridge and cupboards.

As dawn broke one summer's day, I, in my semi-intoxicated state, started to feel increasingly sick. At first I blamed beer from the previous evening. Then it became apparent that Tom had smeared his mother's hair with butter as she slept! This was heating up and emitting an awful stink!

Closer inspection of the kitchen revealed that he had gnawed at the cheese, devoured all the yogurts and the contents of the cat bowl. Any form of liquid that could be poured, had been. It was 5.30 in the morning.

The Hyperactive Children's Support Group

Having felt less than enamoured with the 0-19 Team, I set about doing my own research and stumbled across the HCSG on the internet. The following letter shone a light into my darkness.

Dear Sally Bunday, (This is the founder of the group)

I feel compelled to write to you, as with your help I have now got an adorable 4 year old boy whom I now love very much. This was not the case just six months ago...He has gone from being an aggressive, spiteful child with more tantrums in a day than I care to remember, to a loving, affectionate, bright and intelligent little boy - all because of his diet.

Following the advice given in the booklet, we have eliminated the 'culprits' from his diet - mainly 'colours', chocolate, orange and many preservatives. We have occasional 'blips' as we call them, but these are usually caused by M. having foodstuffs that he shouldn't have, through no fault of his own. He now knows what he can and can't have and willingly goes without.

If only I had asked for your help earlier on, I would have avoided the hate and the unrest in the family. I had to have a course of antidepressants and finally gave up my job as a midwife. Life suddenly looks rosy.

I hope you continue your good work. If only people would recognise that this is a major problem and that hyperactive children can be helped.

Many thanks, Mrs A.G. Reading, Berks.

Already, I had recognised that diet could be a factor with Tom's behaviour. He would be particularly awful if I had allowed him to have sweets. An informative magazine article had educated me about food additives, especially in fruit juices and fizzy drinks. His thirst was still immense and I wondered whether there was something sinister in the orange juice he craved. I began to keep a diary to discover any link between everything he consumed and his behaviour. If only it had been that straightforward!

I maintained these diaries for several months before concluding that there wasn't any reliable association. However, I did subscribe to the Hyperactive Children's Support Group and followed all the dietary advice about colourings, flavourings and foods to avoid. There was a wealth of advice on parenting techniques, most of which I was doing anyway. It was reassuring, though, to realise that other mothers had similar problems with their children. The loneliness abated slightly.

However, I had to admit that his behaviour wasn't just 'over-activeness.' It was an endless daily battle in every sense and it showed no signs of abating. Previously, I had hoped that armed with the power of speech, Tom might have been more open to being reasoned with and less frustrated as he would be able to communicate his feelings.

If anything, it was all deteriorating. I took him to the doctor.

As he trashed her surgery, she fired questions at me. "Are you sure he's not just naughty?" She observed as he clambered up onto the examination bed and leapt off it. "Children do typically push their boundaries at his age."

"No." I retrieved him from bouncing up and down on the weighing scales. "He's been like this for a long time."

"Do you think it's worsened since you separated from his dad?" Noticing his interest in her briefcase, she yanked it out of his reach.

I looked at her, bemused as I sank back down. "How could he remember? He was only six months old."

"Maybe he's just energetic," she suggested. We both watched him. He was using the emptied upturned toy box as an aid to climb onto her desk. I sprang up and seized him again.

"Could you be *depressed* Sarah?" She tapped her pen against the side of her face. "That could be why you're finding it tricky to cope."

"I'm definitely not depressed!" I tried to restrain Tom on my knee before he caused any more destruction. "I sometimes get a bit down with it all, like anyone would. I'm finding it difficult to cope because he's such a handful. He doesn't sleep properly. As you can see he never even stops moving." Powerless to keep hold of him, I lowered him back to the floor. "He's biting constantly and his tantrums are horrendous."

"OK," I struggled to hear her above the din he was creating. "I'm going to get a child psychologist to see you both." I felt like cheering as she typed into her computer. "I'm not sure what they'll be able to do. He's still so young. But we can give it a try."

The Child Psychologist

When it eventually took place, the appointment was far from positive. I decided to take Martin with me. I also invited Peter and Elizabeth. I hoped that 'en-masse', we might be more forceful.

Tom catapulted around the antiseptic-smelling room, like a sprung ball in a pinball machine. We all introduced ourselves. The psychologist was a middle-aged woman; she had a worn face and a brisk voice. She began by reading out the doctor's letter.

"I would be grateful if you could advise this lady who has an 'over-active' little boy." She glanced at Tom before continuing. *"I believe she would benefit from advice in controlling his angry outbursts, particularly when in public. He is also prone to biting."* She pulled a face. *"In addition, she has made me aware that she is having toilet-training difficulties with him."*

"So," began the psychologist, pressing the letter into quarters. "What help would you like in particular?"

"Anything and everything! Whatever you can offer!" I smiled, watching as Tom tipped out a box of bricks. She did not smile back.

"I'm really struggling with him. Stop it Tom!" He was hurling the bricks around. "I've brought along the behaviour diaries I've been keeping for a few months." I fished around in my bag. "Can I read you bits of them?"

"Go ahead." The woman relaxed backwards in her chair, a bored expression on her face. "That might be helpful."

I cleared my throat and began reading. *"Just before bed, I caught him smearing poo over his bedroom wall."* The room was silent. I straightened up in my chair.

"Martin took him to the park where he was throwing stones at cars. He tried to wee over another child but she got away." Martin shook his head at the memory.

"Took him to visit a friend. He bit their dog!"

"He bit their dog!" The woman looked flabbergasted and by the look in her eyes, did not believe me either.

I nodded before continuing. *"Put him to bed at eight. Checked on him at nine, he had stripped his bed, emptied his cupboard of* clothes and was wedged behind his bed with books piled on top of him. He finally settled at around 11.15pm."

I peered at the woman.

"Go on."

Taking a deep breath, I flicked forwards several pages. *"Caught him standing on the table, weeing at the TV"*

Peter chuckled but straightened his face in response to my glare.

"Put kitten in freezer," was an entry made by Elizabeth. Another read *"Shut kitten in dustbin."*

Swapping the diary for another one, I read from a randomly opened page. *"At a friend's house, he took her baby daughter's nappy off and was laughing at her bum!"*

"Using a 'swipe' action, swept all my belongings from my dressing table. After I had picked them up, he did it again."

"And again and again and again," Martin interjected. "Sarah, I don't know why you bother to *try* and keep things on your dressing table."

I ignored him. *"Tantrum on bus. He was screaming and trying to bite me then he bolted into road as we got off.* He behaves like that every time we use public transport," I added.

"He sounds like a character!" she smiled now, surveying him. He was trying to climb up the back of Peter's chair.

"What Sarah is trying to get across to you," Martin addressed the woman now. "Is that the examples of behaviour she has given are not isolated incidents." He glanced at me as though seeking my approval that it was ok to speak out about my son in this way. "Every minute of every day, she has her hands full with him. He never, ever stops. He seizes every opportunity to do something as out of the ordinary as possible."

"He *is* only three." The woman seemed to be disregarding his comments. "Also, no disrespect to you, Sarah, but you are young." Her eyes washed over me in appraisal. "It's often hard to manage."

My face burned with indignation. "I'm twenty three, not sixteen! And I've been on my own with him since he was six months! I'm used to it!"

"It's never easy when you're on your own." Her tone was gentle as she ignored my comments too. I was infuriated.

"I think the diaries you've been keeping are a fantastic idea." She pointed to the books in my hand. "There may well be a link between his behaviour and what he is eating. I'm going to send you an appointment to see a dietician to get further advice." Reaching behind, she took a pen and notebook from her desk.

"And that's it?" I felt deflated as I tried to decipher her writing from upside-down.

"There's not a lot I can do." She shrugged dismissively as she dropped her pen. "I just need to take a few details from you so I know where to send the appointment."

I bent to retrieve the pen. Tom had snatched it up. Knowing I wanted it, he screamed and clutched it tighter. When I finally prised it from his grasp he launched himself to the floor hysterically. I gathered him up and tried to sit him on my knee, which he had never liked. Before gaining the power of movement, I had been able to sit him on my knee and cuddle him. But now he arched his back and flayed his arms wildly.

"Try holding him a little tighter," the woman suggested, noticing his reticence. "That's it. Wrap your arms around him and grip him firmly until his temper subsides."

Tom let me know he did not like this by slinging his head backwards into my face. I jerked it out if his way just in time.

"Hold him as firmly as you can," continued the woman, her face hardening slightly as Tom began booting me. "Place your leg, just across his to stop that." In demonstration, she swung one of her legs across the other. After a few moments Tom's anger seemed to ebb out of him.

"That seems to work." She appeared delighted. "If you restrain him in that way, he will begin to learn that *you're* in charge, not *him*. Whenever he is over-active, just hold him securely until the anger goes." She swept her gaze over Martin, Peter and Elizabeth too as if silently advocating this method to them as well. "Once he realises you have got him and he can't do as he wants, he *will* calm down, you'll see."

Perceptions of Others (A "Social Worker")

Martin and I decided to stop for a drink in a beer garden on the way home. It was a gorgeous evening and we both needed to 'de-stress' after the appointment!

As soon as we parked, Tom sprang from the car with the enthusiasm of an animal just released from captivity. We found a seat but instead of enjoying the play equipment, he kept charging towards the gate. I was up and down, repeatedly dragging him back to the table, terrified he would make it to the gate as there was a road nearby. After a while, he tired of this 'game,' and instead, filled his pocket with stones, finding great amusement in chucking them around. People sat near us peered uncomfortably at him, and us. He laughed wildly at my attempts at prevention.

Then, in an unguarded moment, he took a swipe at my drink. There was an ear-splitting crash as the glass shattered on the floor, then a titter of disapproval went up. My face blazed as every eye in the beer garden rested upon me.

"I'll get you another and then we'll get out of here." Martin rose up, glowering at Tom. "And a dustpan and brush."

"I think we should go now......," I began to protest. But he had already vanished inside.

As I tried to gather the larger shards of glass, Tom tried to bolt towards the pub after Martin. Recalling the advice of the psychologist, I raced after him and hauled him back to our table. Dropping him onto my lap, I endeavoured to firmly hold him in the way she had demonstrated. My arms fastened around his arms and upper body. I pressed him close so that he could not throw his head back. Desperately, he kicked his legs as I prayed he would soon calm down. It was taking all my strength to keep hold of him. His face was contorted with rage as he squealed like a piglet facing slaughter.

"What you are doing is *disgusting!*" hissed a woman, who cannot have been any older than me. She surveyed me with her hands resting on her hips and hatred in her eyes.

"W-what?" I relaxed my hold on Tom. I hadn't planned on interference from onlookers.

"I'm a social worker. That's wrong." Her lipsticked top lip curled in disgust. "It's child abuse. Let him go." She bent forwards and touched his arm. "You're hurting him."

"Of course I'm not!" I ascended up to challenge her, balancing Tom on my hip. "I've been shown by a child psychologist how to restrain him. You don't know what you're on about! Mind your own business!" The air was heavy with silence. Everyone around was mesmerised by the spectacle that was unfolding before them.

"You want that child taking off you!" She beckoned two other women to join her. "You cruel bitch!" She began tugging at Tom from behind.

"Get off him!" I tried to maintain my grip on him.

Suddenly, I was hurled to the ground by the two other women. The 'social worker' began booting me in the head. Thud, thud, thud. Howling in pain, I could hear the wails of Tom echoing around me and could only pray that he would not use this opportunity to bolt into the road.

"Get off her!" Urgent footsteps stamped towards me. "Get the hell away from her!" Martin dragged them all off me and they dispersed into the gathered crowd. He pulled me to my feet and towards the car, hauling Tom behind him. I was weeping hysterically. Hot blood drizzled down the side of my face. The pain to my head was agonising but overwhelmingly, I cried with shame.

The Dietician

I was advised by the dietician to look on the internet for help. The appointment was a waste of time. However I found this form:

netmums.com

Shopping List

E Numbers that can cause problems...

Colours
E102 Tartrazine
E104 Quinloine Yellow
E110 Sunset Yellow
E120 Cochineal
E122 Carmoisine
E123 Amaranth
E124 Ponceau 4R
E127 Erythrosine
E128 Red 2G
E131 Patent Blue V
E132 Indigo Carmine
E133 Brilliant Blue
E142 Green S
E150c Ammonia Caramel
E151 Brilliant Black
E155 Brown GT
E160b Annatto
E161g Ganthaxanthin
E173 Amuninium

Preservatives and anti oxidants
E210-219 Benzoic acid, benzoates
E220-228 Sulphur dioxide, sulphites
E230-232 Benzene derivatives
E249-250 Nitrites
E251-252 Nitrates
E280-283 Propionic acid, propionates
EE310-312 Propyl gallate, gallates
E320 Butylated hydroxyanisole
E321 Bytylated hydroxytoluene

Emulsifiers and thickeners
E407 Carrageenan
E413 Targacanth gum
E420 Sorbitol
E421 Mannitol
E430-436 Polyoxyls

Flavour Boosters
E950 Acesulfame-K
E951 Aspartame
E952 Cylclamate
E953 Isomalt
E954 Saccharin
E965-967 Maltitol, Lactitol, Xylitol

Spot the hidden sugar
Sugar can be hard to spot in children's food, as it's called many different things. All the following are forms of sugar, which is only needed in small amounts and offers your child little, except empty calories:

Sucrose, glucose, fructose, maltose, dextrose, fruit syrup, molasses, maltodextrin.

Look for "no added sugar" on the packet. If you can't see that on a label then read the Nutritional Information panel and look under "Carbohydrates - of which Sugar".

Is a food healthy or not?

This is a lot /100g		This is a little /100g
10g	Sugars	2g
20g	Fats	3g
5g	Saturated Fats	1g
0.5g	Sodium (salt)	0.1g
3g	Fibre	0.5g

Journeying

Martin

May 2007 (3 years, 5 months)

I reinstated the receiver, uneasily sensing that my day was about to be hijacked.

"That was the childminder. She's ill."

"Oh great." Sarah stomped into the room, a surge of panic in her eyes. "Today just gets better. I've got to go to work. I don't suppose ……?" Her expression was pitiful.

"Do I have to?" My heart descended with a thud inside my chest.

Her face grew more beseeching. "Oh, alright then." *How could I say no?* But I was silently berating myself for being weak.

After her departure, I decided to take Tom out in the car. It was easier than attempting to fasten him into his buggy, which was a two person job at the best of times! I grabbed a toy and book to keep him entertained for the brief journey.

Within minutes of embarkment he was winding down his window. Before I had chance to stop the car, he had hurled his book through it. Its pages wildly flapped as it was forcibly ejected onto the road. In my rear view mirror I could see it fluttering in the wind as it was run over by oncoming cars.

Moments later, the hairs on the back of my neck stood up as a result of the sudden fast rush of air they had been exposed to. I was horrified to realise he had opened the car door. Slamming the car to a halt, I leapt out. How could I have been so stupid not to have applied the child lock? Heaving a sigh of relief, I set off again. I had just averted an utter catastrophe. I have no idea how I would have explained that one to Sarah? *Oh yes, I was looking after your little boy, the most precious thing in your universe, but he flung himself from my moving car!*

Sadly, I was unable to prevent him from winding down the back window.

"Tom. No!" As we joined a roundabout, he cast out his toy. The car behind me sounded its horn. "No, leave it on!" In my mirror, I noticed he had unclipped his seatbelt. But nothing could prepare me for what came next. In a split second, he leaned out of the open window and released his door from the outside.

How I held onto him with one arm reaching backwards; and the other trying to manoeuvre the car around the roundabout, I will never know. But somehow I did. Pulling over, I then rested for a few moments, trying to compose myself.

Finally we made it to the park. We had bread for the ducks but Tom decided to feed them one of his new shoes instead. In horror, I watched as he flung it over the railing. It hurtled down the fast flowing river before I had chance to find a stick to fish it out! Sarah would go mad! The shoes had set her back a bit.

On the way home, we stopped off at a shop. Obviously, it was necessary to carry a one-shoed Tom. It was zapping my strength to keep hold of him.

Clearly, this was a marvellous opportunity for an outburst to convey his dissatisfaction at the small pack of sweets I had selected for him. He lashed and kicked at me, flailing his limbs wildly. My face was on fire as I paid; the opinionated eyes of fellow shoppers burning into the back of my head.

The tantrum intensified on the journey home. Its full force could be felt through his feet in the back of my seat, accompanied by ear-splitting screams and being winded as he yanked at my seatbelt in temper.

Silently, I vowed that this would be the last time!

The GP (again)

"Is Tom not with you?" The GP peered beyond me as I entered the surgery.

"No, the childminder's got him." I detected relief within her expression.

"What can I do for you Sarah?" She leant towards me.

"It's Tom," I began. "I need something, anything, to slow him down!" I clasped my hands together as though I was praying for help. "He's on the go constantly! I can't take my eyes off him."

"You know we can't give him anything." She shook her head apologetically. "He's still little. It's not as simple as just being able to medicate him."

"But he's wrecking everything. My home, in fact all I've got. He breaks all his own stuff too." I paused as I remembered other information I needed to add. "Then there's the pooing and the biting. I don't know what to do with him – I'm at my wits end!"

"He's still doing that? Have you tried putting him back in nappies?"

"Of course." I laughed incredulously. "He just removes them. He's potty trained for the childminder." I sighed and tuned my face towards the ceiling. "He's just so naughty; I wish I knew what I was doing wrong!"

"I can refer you to the 0-19 Team again," she suggested, an expression of doubt on her face as she awaited my reply. My heart plummeted.

"But they were useless!" I shuddered at the memory. "There must be someone else who can help!"

"It may be a different person this time. Some of the staff can be more helpful than others." She poised her pen, awaiting my go-ahead. "Obviously they all have expertise in various areas of child development."

"Fine then, I'll give it another try."

I left the surgery feeling anything but optimistic.

Different 'Experts' (The 0-19 Team)

September 1997 (3 years, 9 months)

This time I attended alone. Thankfully it was not the same man as before. There were *two* assessors this time. A man and a woman. Feeling apprehensive, I sat down before them.

"How can we help?" The man eventually raised his head from studying a form. I felt mirth erupting as I noticed his huge nose and combed over hair.

"My son is showing severe behaviour problems." Already intimidated, my voice shook. "I think there could be something wrong with him."

"That's a worrying thing for you to be alleging about your little boy," remarked the woman, surveying me in a way that made me feel even more uncomfortable. She appeared close to retirement age with tightly curled hair and spectacles which hung from a chain and rested upon her bosom. "What on earth makes you think that?

I reeled off all the usual information. Sleeping, impulsivity, over activity, biting, soiling and smearing, etc, etc. I was beginning to feel like I had been through it so many times.....

However, they *seemed* to be paying attention. They were making the right noises as I spoke. This spurred me on. They actually seemed sympathetic as I reeled off my experiences. Even the woman.

"Right, lets get a bit of background," she announced, pulling a pen from her bag and accepting a form thrust at her by her colleague. "Is it just you and Tom at home?"

"No, there's my boyfriend, Martin." I flinched as I used the word *boyfriend*. Obviously *husband* would have sounded more respectable.

"And he's Tom's biological father?" She waited for my response with pursed lips.

"Er, no," I stammered. "He's not actually." I fiddled with my necklace.

"I see." She wrote something down. "And how long have you been together?

"Nearly two years." I leaned against the back of my seat, feeling a little more confident. Two years was decent. I was not some mother that just introduced any old man to her son.

"Does he get on with Tom?" The veins and tendons in her neck protruded as she bobbed her head up and down in time to her questions.

"Of course." For a moment I wished he had accompanied me to this meeting. "But he struggles with his behaviour too."

"How old was Tom when you separated from his real dad?" She turned her form over.

"About six months." It seemed such a long time ago.

"Hmmmm. Right." Looking thoughtful, she uncrossed her legs. "Parental separation might be a contributory factor here. It often is."

"But he was six months old! And it was all perfectly amicable. His dad still sees him. I don't think it's that at all!" A snort of laughter escaped from within me.

The man addressed me next. "What about your parents Sarah? Do they help out?" He fired questions without waiting for a response. "Does Tom have a good relationship with them?"

I shook my head. "I don't have any contact with my mum, to be honest." Holding my breath, I knew this was probably the vital nugget of information they would have been waiting for.

"Oh." The woman looked taken aback. "Why's that?"

"Well, I used to be in care." My voice was unsteady. "It's a long time ago now, but I didn't see my family at all for eight years." Every time I spoke the words aloud, it provoked a tug of sadness within me. "I'm in touch with them now though, apart from my mum, that is."

The man and woman swapped glances. "*You were in care?* For how long?"

"Why do you want to know?" I sat forward, poised to defend my corner.

"It could be relevant." The woman appeared positively gleeful at my revelation. "These things often are."

"Just whilst I was in my teens. But it wasn't my fault," I added quickly. This was what I had fretted about. That they would blame *me* for Tom's behaviour.

"Have you any brothers or sisters?"

"Two sisters. Two brothers. All younger." I pressed my hands together in my lap.

"Were *they* in care with you?" The woman was continuously scribbling as she quizzed me.

"No. Why?" Butterflies were batting their wings defensively within my stomach. "What does that matter anyway?"

"Why were only *you* in care?" The woman seemed to be relishing my discomfort.

"Because it was only me that my mum didn't want." Inwardly, I cringed, aware of how pathetic I sounded. "She wasn't well at the time."

"What was the matter with her?" *Nosy cow!*

"Severe depression." I studied the gaudy floral lightshade above my head intently. "She was in hospital for a while."

"Depression can be hereditary." Pausing her writing, she seemed to examine me. "Have you ever suffered from it, Sarah?"

"I thought we were here to discuss Tom." My usual composure was starting to slip away from me.

"Yes, but it's always fascinating to know what issues parents might be bringing from their own childhoods." The man spoke again. They were clearly preaching from the same handbook. "It can affect how they nurture *their* children." His hesitation indicated that he was possibly uncertain of whether to proceed with his next remark. But he expressed it anyway. "History *does* have a way of replicating itself, you know."

"What are you implying?" The hairs on the back of my neck seared up.

"Nothing yet, but we do have to ascertain the facts."

My eyes raised skyward. "The fact is that I'm here to get help and support for my little boy." My voice was sharp now. "Why are you harping on about my childhood? I'm nothing like my own mum. I'm a caring mother and love my son. Otherwise I wouldn't be here!"

They both studied me quietly.

"I'm not sure what assistance we can offer you." The man was obviously startled by my tone. "He is very young. Parenting has a huge impact on behaviour…"

I jumped to my feet as his voice trailed off.

"I'm not going to sit here while you dig for dirt." I strode towards the door and yanked at the handle. "You're not going to help me, are you? You're just looking for someone to blame." Banging the door of the oppressive little room, I hurtled towards the freedom of the car park, vowing to soldier on myself. *What the hell did they know anyway?*

And I did, for a while, as best as I could. But I knew eventually, we would have to be taken seriously. I had finally admitted to myself that there was something behaviourally and emotionally not right with Tom. It was probably something simple to treat too. I just needed someone to listen to me.

5th October 1997

Dear Sarah,

Please accept this letter as notice that I am unable to continue having your son, Tom, in my charge.

As we have discussed on many occasions, the problems with him biting and bullying other children are becoming more serious, to the point where other parents are making threats to remove their children from my care if I do not sort out the situation.

In addition to this, as we are both aware, Tom is having a terrible impact on the other children's behaviour with his recent habit of swearing.

As you know, I am sympathetic to your difficult circumstances and because of this; I am willing to give you two weeks notice in order that you can make alternative arrangements.

I hope you can understand my predicament.

Yours, Sharon

Requirements of a Suitable Day Nursery

1. High and impossible-to-climb perimeter fencing or walling.
2. Bolted exterior doors.
3. A willingness to keep behaviour and food diaries.
4. A menu that is free of food additives and e-numbers.
5. Robust furniture and play equipment.
6. Staff with a sense of humour.
7. Staff who are eternally vigilant.
8. Staff who are sympathetic to the plight of mothers trying to cope with a 'challenging' child.

An Exit Strategy

Martin

Tom was at his worst on a morning. The breakfast throwing and refusals to dress were nothing new. But he had devised a *new* tactic. It was as though he were trying everything in his power to make mornings as problematic as he could.

I was powerless to intervene as Sarah repeated the same procedure with him day-after-day as she got ready to go to work. I would cringe as the same question was asked:

"Do you need the toilet before we go Tom?"

He would shake his head, a devilish grin dancing upon his lips.

"Are you sure? Will you just have a little try for mummy?"

"No! Don't need to go!"

From the armchair which faced towards the hallway and the front door, my gaze would veer back and forth from Sarah, dashing about, to Tom, unusually in one place; pressed up against the front door. If you watched him carefully enough, you would notice the bent legs and the strain on his face. By then it was too late to halt the inevitable.

"Oh Tom!" Sarah would shriek, inhaling the stench. "I asked if you needed to go!"

He would stare at her, a mixture of innocence and mirth, as she prepared to remove his soiled clothes and replace them with clean ones. Every single morning.

The Extended Family

"Don't laugh at him," I would implore my brothers, amused at his antics, particularly his swearing. To hear such dreadful words emerging from such a little and as many would say, "angelic-looking" boy; was shocking. I have no idea where he had witnessed them, but he used them repeatedly.

It was doubly mortifying when I was out with him. On public transport, I would silently pray that he would not have an outburst! To make it worse, he would thrive on the stunned reaction from his audience.

My brothers and my stepdad visited every week and Tom would become more and more manic as the evening wore on. Never did one of these visits occur without one sort of breakage or another. It might just be a cup or a picture. At others, it was something more awkward. There was the time he swung from the curtains, pulling the whole rail down; and another when he yanked one of the doors from the TV cabinet.

My family would eventually tire of his behaviour. There is only so long that anyone can endure an overactive three-year-old leaping all over them!

"You *dirty* little git!" Alan, my stepdad, wrenched Tom into the air and held him aloft, as he carted him towards his bedroom. Alan then vanished into the bathroom.

"What happened?" We all whispered to each other. "Did anyone see?"

It transpired that Tom had clambered onto the sofa, lodged himself behind Alan's back and weed over him. Stephen and Chris howled with laughter as they learned what had enraged Alan.

Chris, however, was not laughing later when Tom weed in his coffee!

Humiliation

January 1998 (4 years, 1 month)

It was not long before I was hauled into the office at nursery whilst I collected Tom. It was a stark room; devoid of any indication that it was linked to a nursery, apart from a child's painting on the back of the door.

"We need to speak to you about his behaviour," stated the officer-in-charge, pointing to a chair in front of her desk.

Sighing, I sat down. *Here we go.*

"Other parents are beginning to complain." She looked directly into my face, her hands clasped together on the table before her.

"What's he done?" I tried to disguise the weariness in my voice.

"He's constantly swearing and bullying others, often smaller children." She paused and seemed to be searching my expression for a reaction. "He doesn't seem to have any concept of sharing when he's here. He actually becomes violent when he wants to play with something. Is he like this at home? Does he have any brothers or sisters?"

"No, it's just him." I could feel my face firing up. "I do have friends with children of a similar age that he plays with though. He *is* used to playing with others."

"Does he play considerately with them?" She didn't wait for my answer. "I ask because he seems to be having real difficulty mixing with others *here.* When he does occasionally strike a partnership with another child, he becomes controlling and possessive. He certainly cannot play with more than one child at a time."

"I thought he'd settle here, surrounded by different children; especially the older ones. There's so much to occupy him too." I felt a bit guilty then that I had not mentioned a word about Tom's behavioural problems when I had enrolled him. But I had been scared of being refused a place. "I do have problems with him at home as well, I know I should have mentioned them before but I thought he'd improve here. I'll try to speak to him about what you've said to me, if I can get him to listen, that is!"

"Well, if you could *try* to speak to him, we'd be grateful."

"I'll do my best." I started to rise from my seat, thinking the conversation had concluded. But she continued.

"We're having difficulties when he plays outside too." I sank back down. "His climbing ability is extraordinary."

I laughed. "I know."

She didn't laugh. She just continued. "He keeps trying to scale the exterior fence and today got onto the roof of the kitchen." She gestured through the window to indicate the roof she was referring to. "He doesn't seem to have any concept of height. None of us have ever seen anything like it!"

"He's always climbed." I was not shocked when I looked out at the roof. Or when I noticed the height of the fence. "He's climbed from when he could move! He has no sense of danger whatsoever."

"Well, it looks like we're going to have to maintain our vigilance!" She stopped, again making me think she had finished. "Oh, while I'm thinking about Tom, do you have any problems at home with mealtimes."

"Well, yes," I relied hesitantly. "But he's getting *slightly* better."

"Well, you'll have to let us into your secret." She glanced through the interior window to where the children were sitting down to an afternoon snack. A member of staff was sat beside Tom, evidently keeping him in check. "It's getting to the point where we may have to separate him from the others at lunchtime. He's a terrible influence. There's more on the floor than he's eating. He's unable to concentrate."

I kept nodding as I listened to her.

"He seems to have an unlimited supply of energy. We'd expect him to be burning himself out by lunchtime with the level of activity he maintains. Most of our three-year-olds have a nap after lunch."

"Tom's never needed much sleep. Not even when he was tiny."

The officer-in charge shook her head as she carried on. "I should also mention his tendency to do his toileting outside. Tom has no qualms whatsoever about just pulling down his pants and weeing wherever the mood takes him. When he needs the toilet, he should be telling one of us." Her expression was grim. "It's unacceptable."

"I agree," I sighed. "It's just a phase he's going through at the moment. I hope to God it soon passes." There was no other way forward: it was time to be honest. Maybe they could help me if I was. "I don't know what to do with him. The doctor and health visitor have seen us on numerous occasions; we've been to the 0-19 Team twice, a dietician *and* a child psychologist!"

"That information should have been disclosed when you enrolled him with us."

"I was worried you wouldn't take him."

She did not answer; I accepted her silence as a sign that my initial fears were justified. Our conversation concluded with an agreement that they would collaborate in monitoring Tom and maintain records of his diet and behaviour. Monthly review meetings would be held to discuss his progress.

With a pain in my head beginning to emerge, I scuttled from the office to retrieve him from the snack table.

"No!" He bolted inn the direction of the toilets. "Go away!"

My face was on fire. "Don't be silly Tom!" Other parents were observing in astonishment. "It's time to go home." I dashed after him.

"Get off me! Don't like you!" He tried to yank himself away from the grip I had on his arm. I'm staying here!"

The familiar sting of tears stabbed behind my eyes, which I kept fixed on his defiant face. "Come on sweetheart." I could not bear to see anyone else's expression. "You can come back tomorrow!"

In the end I had to practically drag him out. In his eyes, home was probably boring; compared to nursery, anyway.

Hauling him in the direction of the bus stop, I could hardly stand to speak to him. I cannot imagine what the staff and other parents must have made of us. This behaviour recurred on several occasions as I collected him; it was also inflicted on Martin who immediately vowed he would never pick him up again!

On the bus ride home did Tom:

a. Pull my hair?
b. Bite my hand?
c. Scratch the side of my face?
d. Wail and thrash uncontrollably?
e. Throw his shoe at a man four seats in front of us?
Or f. All of the above?

(You guessed it!)

Suspension from the Day Nursery

Soon after, the officer-in-charge summoned me to her office again. I was accustomed to regular negative reports, usually relayed from the nursery nurses. This was the second time I had been called into the office.

"I'm not sure what action we're going to take," she advised me grimly, as she leant on her desk. "But Tom has severely bitten a younger child."

"Oh no!" I took a sharp intake of breath as I accepted the seat she pointed to. "I don't know what to say! I'm so sorry!"

"She was laid in her carry cot after lunch," she continued, "and Tom, must have realised that no one was watching, so he bit her thumb as she was falling asleep. Her thumb has actually blackened with the injury. She's not even a year old."

I gasped. I was horrified. "Was it definitely him who did it?" My voice trailed off. It's just you said no one was ……"

"The guilt was written all over his face." Her mouth was set in a thin, hard line. "I think even Tom was taken aback by her screams. Her mother is furious as I'm sure you can appreciate."

"Can you tell her how sorry I am? I really am." I was on the brink of tears.

"I think it would be in everyone's interests if you were to collect Tom and leave the building before the baby's mother has the opportunity to confront you." Her eyes were fixed on the office door as she spoke to me. "Understandably, she is making all kinds of threats. Tom will have to be kept away from nursery for the remainder of the week. We have to be seen to be taking action."

The door burst open then. The entrant needed no introduction.

"You're monster of a boy!" she shrieked as she stormed towards me. "Have you seen what he's done to my baby?"

"I'm sorry!" I sprang up from my chair. "I'm so sorry!"

"His teeth want extracting!" she snarled as I crept past her. "What an animal!"

Hardly daring to meet her eyes, I slipped out of the room. I had never felt shame like it in all my life.

Starting School

January 1999 (4 years, 9 months)

"Come on Tom. You've got to get some sleep." I twisted my head around Tom's door. It was nearly midnight and I was about to turn in myself. "You've got a big day tomorrow."

"Can't get to sleep," he muttered from beneath his bed. "My brain won't stop thinking."

"It's just because you're excited about big school." I reached under his bed to ease him from his hiding place.

"Never can get to sleep," he groaned. "Lots of spiders keep wiggling inside me."

"You'll be fine once you get used to school. It will *make* you tired."

Martin joined me on Tom's first day. Together we observed as he hurtled around the playground. Unfortunately he was too preoccupied with looking around at the other boys to concentrate on his own direction, therefore went flying over a bench, crashing his head into the ground at the other side.

"Oh my God!" I rushed to his side as blood seeped out of his forehead. A crowd immediately gathered around us, only dispersing as a whistle was blown.

"Trust Tom to make an entrance on his first day," I smiled at his new teacher, Mrs Henderson, as I led him into his new classroom, clutching paper towels to his head.

"We'll keep an eye on him," she assured me. "Now Tom, what do you like to do most?"

"Draw," he replied without hesitation. "And climb."

"I don't think there'll be any climbing today." She passed him some paper and a tin of crayons. "But perhaps your mummy would like you to draw her a picture. You can give it to her when she comes back for you."

That was my cue to leave him. I had every faith, in any case, that 'big school', would help solve many of our problems. It would tire him out, and provide him with some much-needed structure and further discipline.

The first few weeks passed without incident until one afternoon, I was waiting beside the clique of mothers for the end-of-day bell when my thoughts were broken into by the shrill voice of his class teacher.

"I need to chat with you about his behaviour," Mrs Henderson began, as she bustled me inside the classroom where Tom seemed settled on a chair with a book. "We're having a few problems, unfortunately. He's not getting on well with many of the other children. When they won't be his partner, he hits them."

"And that's not all!" boomed Mrs Armstrong, the head teacher, striding into the classroom and coming up behind Mrs Henderson. "Tom is the *only* child I have *ever* had from Reception class sent to my office."

"W-why?" I stammered.

"Going to the toilet in the playground! The lunchtime assistants say he is always doing it. We've had a chat about it already, haven't we Tom?" He slunk down in his chair as she addressed him directly. "You know we don't do such disgusting things at school!" She looked at me then.

"I'll speak to him," I promised.

"Are you going to tell your mum what else you did today Tom?" His teacher, in a gentler tone, nodded first towards him then the fish tank."

"I wasn't going to hurt them." His voice was small. "I just wanted to see what would happen if they weren't in the water."

"We'll have to find somewhere else for you to sit if you can't be trusted near the fish tank," she continued sternly. "Have *you* got any pets Tom?"

"A cat. She's called Lulu."

"And how would you feel if anyone was to hurt her like you nearly did with the fish?"

I prevented myself from informing them of the necessity to protect Lulu from him. In recent weeks it had been necessary to rescue her from being trapped in the door and more seriously, shut in the freezer. Only the previous Sunday, I had stopped him as he was trying to lower her into the bath.

"Sad," Tom replied, without averting his eyes from his book.

The Enemy Within

"He says he's not got any toys at home," Tom's teacher informed me on another occasion day after school. She had again asked me to stay behind for a word. "Although that doesn't give him permission to steal toys from school."

"Of course he's got toys." My face blazed as I glared to where Tom was scaling the racks in the cloakroom. "Well, what remains that he hasn't yet destroyed yet."

Unlike most parents, it was a relief that Christmas was approaching again. For several months, I had been saving to present him with yet another batch of toys.

Martin thought I was crazy. "They'll all be broken within a month." Condescendingly, he watched as I wrapped the carefully chosen toys. "Then he'll be going round trying to get people to feel sorry for him again."

It was not just toys he destroyed. The next day when I collected him after school, he had obviously been left unattended with scissors. A chunk of his hair was missing, there was a huge hole in his jumper and he had unpicked the stitching from one of his shoes.

These were not isolated events; all his clothes, shoes and toys had a restricted shelf life; much more limited than those given to kids of a similar age.

Christmas arrived and departed with the usual levels of angst and destruction.

I embraced Tom's first day back at school in the New Year with gratitude. At the time, my youngest brother Stephen was staying with us.

"I'm not going," Tom asserted as he observed Stephen playing the games console. "I'm staying here with Stephen. You can't make me go to school."

"Oh yes I can!" I marched towards Tom, grabbed hold of his arm and hauled him to his feet.

With challenging eyes, he glared at me as he swore and rammed his fist against the wall. Stephen shook his head.

"I'd have been murdered if I'd carried on like that at his age!" Putting the controller down, he switched off the TV.

"Get to your room!" I grabbed Tom's hand and pulling him towards the door. "Don't you dare come out until Liz gets here!"

Liz was the *latest* childminder, employed three days a week to collect and deliver him to school; enabling me to work.

Tom slammed the living room door with every fragment of strength he possessed. I jumped as his bedroom door was also banged.

"I can't believe how strong he is for a six-year-old," remarked Stephen, retrieving the controller.

"I know," Sinking into a chair, my heart sank with me as I contemplated the enormity of my day-after day, week-after-week; month-after-month struggle for survival. I had given up trying to get any professional help with him. I was on my own.

"Oh my God, what have you done?" Worriedly, I peered at Tom as he re-entered the room moments later with several visible scratch marks to his neck.

"He's actually made himself bleed! Why have you done it mate?" Stephen's worried gaze transported itself from me, back to Tom.

"I told her I wasn't going to school." He swaggered across the room. "And now I can't. Not with my neck like this." Throwing himself on the sofa next to Stephen, his expression was as smug as a guilty robber who's got away with it.

A car beeped its horn outside.

"Get your coat on." I hurled it towards him.

"No. I'm not going!" Folding his arms, he sat as far back on the sofa as he could.

"Now!" I started towards him.

In a fit of temper, he ripped the hood from his coat then fled back to his bedroom, again slamming the door. I raced outside to where Liz waited, with her other three charges in the back. Tom normally travelled in the front with her so he couldn't bully anyone.

"Where is he?" With a puzzled face, she wound her window down.

"Having one hell of a tantrum!" My voice was trembled with stress. "Because my brother is staying with us, Tom's refusing to go to school. He's even scratched his neck in temper."

"He hasn't, has he?" Liz climbed out of the car. Actually, I wanted to have a bit of a chat with you about his behaviour. There's been a few problems with him at ...."

We were distracted as Stephen suddenly appeared, hauling Tom behind him.

"If he goes to school without any more carrying on, I've promised we'll have a game on the play station at home time," Stephen announced, jubilantly.

"What possessed you to that to your neck?" Liz looked astonished.

"She made me!" Tom wagged an accusing finger towards me.

A feeling of liberation swept over me as the car containing Tom eventually pulled away, leaving me free to set off for work. But there was a call for me shortly after arriving there.

"Is that Tom's mum?" It was the head from his school, whose voice I had grown too familiar with!

"Yes, is there a problem?" None of my colleagues were around to listen in, for which I felt grateful.

"I'm afraid so." She paused for a moment. "I'm afraid Tom has made a rather serious allegation against you............he's disclosed to our caretaker that you're responsible for the scratch marks on his neck."

"W-what! Of course I'm not!" I was incandescent with fury. "He did them himself this morning, carrying on over not wanting to come to school!"

"He did it himself?" Doubt trickled through her words.

"Yes, you've got to believe me! I'd never do anything like that!" Jumping from my chair, I checked along the office corridor that no one could overhear my conversation. "He's lying!"

"Did anyone else see him do it?"

"No, not exactly, but my brother was in the house at the time and knows what happened! And my childminder!" I was garbling; terrified. "She'll back me up as well!" *How could I be getting blamed for this?*

I rang Martin and wept hysterically down the phone.

"Get on the phone to the childminder NOW!" There was more anger than worry in his words. "This needs bloody sorting!"

Her number was constantly engaged. Pacing up and down the office, I glanced out of the window. It was a glistening winters' day and people were scurrying around their business. I felt different to them all; burdened and blamed. *Thank God the boss had not been in with any of this going on!* I hit the redial button again.

"Liz it's Sarah," I announced, feeling weak with gratitude that she had finally picked up.

"I thought I'd hear from you soon."

"I need you to talk to Tom's school for me?" Nervously, I twisted the phone wire within my fingers. "He's told them I scratched his neck!"

"They've been in touch already." Her voice was calm, unlike mine. "Don't worry, I've put them straight."

"What did you say?"

"That you would *never* hurt him, and that he admitted in front of me how he'd scratched *himself*."

"Thanks Liz." I sank back into my chair. "I've been worried they would believe him."

"He's a little so-and-so isn't he? What a dreadful thing to say."

"I know." *What a kick in the teeth.* I felt utterly deflated.

Within days Liz presented me with her notice. She avoided my gaze as she told me. "I'll hang onto him till you sort something else out."

It was decent of her, considering. He had tried pinching things from her house and swearing at the other children. The only option left was to hand *my* notice in at work and search for a job nearer home so I could just work during school hours.

Two days later she had only just collected him from me when she rang.

"Do you know that Tom has got £23 on him?"

"No……. where's he got that from?" Then, as I rummaged for my purse, I realised. I tipped it up. Empty.

"It's mine," I informed her, miserably. "Can you take it off him? And keep an eye on your handbag whilst he's at your house later."

Six years old and thieving money from me! If he can do that now; what's he going to be capable of when he's older?

The Behaviour Chart – 1st Attempt

Soon after, we moved from the flat that had been our home for over six years. Our new house had a little yard at the front and was huge inside.

Tom progressed from his box room to having an ample bedroom with a skylight. I bought a loft bed for him, rugs, cushions and posters. The adjacent 'spare' room housed his TV and my ironing pile Here he could watch films and play his games console to his heart's content.

At the time of the move, he became unsettled. The cutting of his clothes and chunks of his hair became more frequent. On hearing the word 'no' he would grit his teeth and nip his own skin until it reddened. When angry, he thumped himself in the face and would lash out at my attempts to restrain him. His sleeping deteriorated too. From being asleep by midnight, it became one in the morning or beyond. At the time, I attributed it to the upheaval of the house move.

That month when I got paid I stuffed a bag with pocket money sized treats; felt-tips, cars, bouncy balls, balloons, that sort of thing. Then I devised a behaviour chart. He had to get a tick next to each 'criteria' to choose from the 'treat bag' each day:

Getting ready for school with no fuss in morning; good behaviour at school; eating dinner without misbehaving, etc. If he managed to get six treats in the week then he could choose an outing: swimming, the cinema, bowling, or somewhere else within reason.

For the first few days I tried to overlook bad behaviour just so I could give him a tick. When it could not be ignored; he limbered up to the high kitchen shelf and stole his reward.

A 'Break' Away

"We're going to have a holiday at the Lake District," I informed Tom as we loaded the car up. "We'll be sleeping in a tent!"

Martin and I were intending to have a few days there later that year, for our honeymoon, so we wanted to 'test drive' the place first.

The journey felt eternal.

"Tom, quit doing that!" Martin glanced in his rear view mirror. Poking his fingers down his throat, Tom was trying to make himself retch.

"That's disgusting! Stop it!" But it was too late. He threw up all over the back seat.

"Maybe it was car sickness," I grimaced as I dabbed at his slimy vomit with kitchen towel. As usual, I was defending him.

"Like hell it was!" Michael recoiled at the pungent mess. "I saw exactly what he was doing."

When we eventually arrived, Tom vaulted from the car, straight towards the campsite shop.

"Sweets!" he demanded, without pausing for a response.

"You must be joking." I ferreted around in my bag for our booking form. "You were sick on the way here!"

"I did it on purpose." He halted at the entrance of the shop and surveyed me jubilantly. He obviously expected to have sweets if he wasn't *really* ill.

"What did I tell you?" Martin's face bore a smug expression as he slid out of the car. "There's no way he's getting any sweets!"

"Yes I am!" Tearing into the shop, he grabbed a packet and slammed them on the counter. I marched in behind him.

"Sorry." I snatched them away from the shopkeeper. "He's not allowed them. I'll pop them back."

Tom then screeched the worst swear word in his repertoire as he hurled himself to the ground. Flouncing out of the shop, I left him there. He sprang up and raced after me.

"I want sweets!" He was wailing as though he had never been fed as he booted the sign outside the shop with such force that it wobbled over. The shopkeeper followed us out. His hands were thrust into his apron pockets, as he shook his head, no doubt denouncing my parenting skills.

Because he was physically refusing to put one foot in front of the other, I half dragged Tom, half carried him towards the spot where Martin had begun to pitch our tent. Hiss attention was suddenly diverted towards an adventure playground. Wrenching himself free, he bolted in its direction.

"Not so fast!" Hurtling after him, I caught hold of the hood on his jacket.

"But mum, it's ace!" His previous tantrum seemed to have been forgotten by him.

"You don't deserve to be playing in the park." I peered across to where Martin had begun unloading the car. "Not after the way you've carried on today."

However, I gave in. He was in my vision from the spot where we were assembling the tent, battling against the wind. It was a tougher fight against Tom though when I attempted to retrieve him. By the time we returned to our pitch, Martin had lit a barbecue.

"Here, have a drink." I handed Tom some juice. As a kneejerk reaction, he tipped it over the barbecue, which sizzled violently in response, flames becoming smoke. Satisfaction crept across Tom's face at the power he had yielded.

"You little ....!" Martin looked ready to explode alongside the spitting embers. "I don't even know why we bothered coming!"

*   *   *

There was a notable absence at my wedding. For me, it gaped like a crevice.

The year before Tom had been a page boy for a friend. On that very day, I had declared that I would not be exposing myself to the same predicament.

At the start of the day, Tom had looked adorable in his suit and cravat. Initially though, he refused to enter the church after the bride. After I had spent several minutes begging and bribing him, he had agreed, only to cause uproar once inside.

I had been forced to drag him out again, therefore missed my friend's ceremony and was forced instead to peripherally listen to the echo of their chosen hymns from the churchyard.

None of their photos featured Tom. Scaling gravestones and climbing trees was a preferable activity. Eventually, he ensnared the other page boy and bridesmaid too. By the reception they all looked like the children of Steptoe!

"Why *anyone* would want Tom as a page boy is beyond me!" Martin had snorted as we sat observing Tom catapult around the other dancers on the dance floor.

Even though I knew it would cause carnage, I would have given my right arm to choose him as my page boy. But we knew that our big day would become his. I wrestled with the dilemma until eventually Martin took it out of my hands.

"He's not coming." His tone confirmed the matter was not up for discussion. "He'll ruin it if he's there. In fact if *he's* there, I won't be!"

Eventually we reached a compromise and agreed he could be at the reception. But we firstly allocated specific people to help keep an eye on him.

A Sibling for Tom

April 2001 (7 years, 3 months)

How I will know that my second baby is different from my first:
1. The baby will be calm when born, not crimson and 1screaming its lungs out.
2. The baby will settle when lifted for a cuddle.
3. The baby will sleep.
4. It will only need milk every few hours.
5. His or her cry won't be a highly pitched screech.
6. The baby will be relaxed, no thrashing arms and legs.
7. It will be soothed when on hearing my voice.

I pray, I pray, I pray.
No way can I go through it all again.

Parents Evening

May 2001 (7 years, 5 months)

Despite extending the invitation, nobody would accompany me to parent's evening!

I wrestled with the door at the school's entrance against the wind and was comforted by the blast of warm air that greeted me. Immediately, I was escorted back in time by the dusty wooden aroma combined with rubbery plimsoll. Raking my fingers through my windswept hair, I tried to tidy it in order to present myself as a 'respectable' parent. Then I waited outside the classroom.

Leafing through his maths and English books that had been left there, it was slightly heartening to notice that when he had attempted to do some work, most of it had been marked correct. But disappointingly, much of the time, he would be lucky just to jot down the date and the title. Sometimes he may have answered one or two questions or written a sentence. His whole book was scrawled over in red pen: *not enough work Tom, must try harder Tom, this is not good enough: please see me.*

As I continued to wait, my gaze landed upon his class photo pinned to the classroom door. I scanned the faces for Tom. Of course! There he was! Displaying a fiendish grin, he had been positioned next to the teacher.

Laughter rang out from within the classroom. A clock ticked impatiently. *How much longer?* I wanted to get this over with. I searched the corridor walls for Tom's artwork but couldn't find any. The wind, rattling through the crumbly walls, made me tremble slightly. It was eerie being in the school so late at night.

The classroom door eventually burst open and two deliriously happy parents emerged. It must have been good news for them.

"Come in." Mr Murphy held the door wide for me. "Have a seat."

Creeping into the classroom like a timid child, I then sat down as directed. My gaze remained downcast; there was no way it could meet his. My eyes struggled to adjust to the fluorescent lighting after the dinginess of the corridor. As I prepared myself for the onslaught, my heart rate accelerated.

"Well," he began. "Firstly thanks for coming in. I'm not sure where to start. Let's begin with some positives." Sitting bolt upright, he avoided eye contact with me.

Positives! These I was interested in hearing!

"Firstly, his punctuality and attendance are good," he stated as he referred to a chart that sat before him. "And he's certainly a lively member of the class. Mostly a little *too* lively though."

I laughed nervously. He did not laugh. Or even smile.

"Are there any problems or issues at home that might be affecting him?" Now he met my eyes directly. I quickly looked away.

"We've moved house." I shuffled uncomfortably on the tiny chair. "That's not had a good effect on his behaviour."

"I know about that. But he's gone downhill considerably at school. Is there anything else?"

"He's going to be getting a brother or sister." My hand inadvertently flew to my swollen belly.

"That can unsettle children though not usually to *this* degree. There's nothing else?"

I shook my head. "I would've let you know if there was."

"It's just his conduct is like nothing I've ever seen." He looked troubled as he continued. "He can be, forgive me for putting it like this, well *wild.*"

"I know," My voice was faint. "It's the same for me at home. I can't do a thing with him."

He frowned. "I gather you've had him to one or two specialists."

"One or two," In spite of my nerves, I chuckled. "And some. Not one of them had been able to help."

"It's not good for him and it's certainly not fair on the rest of the class. No one learns a thing. I've started segregating him and making him work *there.*" He gestured towards a small table right in front of his own desk. "But even when parked there, right under my nose, he still manages to cause extreme disruption. So then we shift his table into the corridor." He pointed towards the door.

"Meaning my teaching assistant is also leaving the room to supervise him. It can't go on!"

"I'm sorry." I yearned to be anywhere else but in front of this teacher.

"You *must* try to speak to him." His voice had an urgent edge to it. "It's getting to the point where we might have to bring in outside assistance." Reaching into a folder, he produced a form which he thrust towards me. "If this ends up being the case, do we have your consent to proceed?"

"Of course.....I only hope you have more success than I have. Glancing down the form, I accepted the pen he offered. "Where do I need to sign?"

"Just there." He pointed. "We can only try. There's no way we can continue as we have been doing."

"The more he gets to know someone, the worse he behaves. You've probably noticed that yourself." I gained a sense that this particular teacher did not seem to be talking down or blaming me, which helped me relax. "It's been the case with *all* his teachers, childminders and even when he used to go to nursery. To begin with, he's wary of people but that diminishes as soon as he realises what buttons to press and where weaknesses lie in others."

The conversation moved onto the usual renditions of Tom's conduct in school: fighting, spitting, swearing, stealing and urinating in the playground.

Upon exiting the classroom, I realised a backlog of parents had accrued. I dared not meet anybody's condescending gaze as I traipsed past them.

No wonder no one had wanted to come with me to parents evening!

Looking after Tom

Elizabeth

December 2001 (7 years, 11 months)

As Sarah progressed through her pregnancy, Tom inevitably spent more time with us. One afternoon, I arrived home and was taken aback to discover him playing calmly, alone in the garden.
"What are you doing?" I peered at his careful structures in the soil.
"Making a graveyard." He was engrossed in his activity. "Look, those are the graves. That's a car with the body in, this is a coffin."
"Oh." I studied the mounds he had formed. "Do you not want to play a more *cheerful* game?"
His games were bizarre. Boxes became coffins for his soft toys. His pictures depicted guns, graves or violence. As at his mum's, we were vigilant in not allowing him to encounter any violent viewing; however that did not seem to prevent these 'games.'
We had started to allow him to play outside. By now, he was almost eight and would play on the expanse of grass adjacent to our home. I could keep him in vision from the balcony of our first floor flat. He and a neighbouring boy of a similar age would seek each other out. But Tom would want to play fighting games and the other boy didn't. Tom would try to control the play so inevitably their time together was usually fleeting.
Some older boys once invited him to join their game of football. I remember thinking how positive this might be. However, he attempted to dominate the game and refused to pass the ball to anyone else! He was soon ejected!
"His swearing's getting out of hand again," Sarah informed me as I collected him the following week. "One of the neighbours has complained and decided Tom can't play with her son again."
"I'll keep an eye on that then," I sighed, accepting a bag of his clothes from her.

"Oh and unfortunately, he can't ride his bike at yours this week." She nodded towards where it lay, forlornly in the garden. "He's wrecked it in temper. It had a puncture and I didn't know how to fix it. He's repeatedly thrown it at the wall." She continued to stare at it, sadly. "I could see him from the window, flattening it. It's buckled now!"

That evening, Tom tantrummed wildly because he wanted his bike! After a while, Peter ordered him to his room. We curled up together on the sofa, watching a film and were engrossed that it was a while before we acknowledged the absolute silence.

"Go and see what he's up to love." Peter hit the pause button on the remote.

When I checked in his room I noticed that he had scrawled all over one of his walls and his duvet cover with felt tip pens. Stuffing from his soft toys was strewn across every surface. Most of them had had their heads torn off and Tom was now busy yanking out the remaining stuffing.

Tom's stay became extended because Sarah ended up in hospital having the baby. She escaped the two phone calls we received from school.

On Monday we were informed that other parents had marched into school to complain about him as he had been bullying their son. Then on Tuesday he absconded after flying into a rage because he had not got his chosen part in the school play. They had even reported his departure to the police! Luckily he resurfaced soon after in a nearby park.

A Time for Calm

I was mindful of the fact that older siblings can feel sidelined when a new baby comes along. For this reason I had bought Tom a present and a card saying *You're a Big Brother Now!* I had it ready to give to him when Elizabeth brought him to the hospital to meet little Alex.

I studied his face for a reaction. He looked shyly at me as I sat, propped up in the hospital bed. Then he astounded me. "I know how you got a baby……..you did sex." He grinned.

Elizabeth and I exchanged uncomfortable glances as his attention switched to his new brother. "Do you want to hold him?" I offered, as I started to manoeuvre myself from the bed.

Nodding, he launched himself into the spot from which I had just emerged. I gently passed Alex to him. Then watched. I still smile at the photograph capturing that moment. Tom leaned like a statue against my pillows, cradling his little brother, protectively resting his hand under his head as though he was the most precious thing in the world. The pride is evident in his expression and I recall the surge of hope that everything was going to turn out fine.

Alex turned out to be the complete opposite of Tom. I knew he was different as soon as he was born. A contented baby, he adored his sleep and even when awake, would just lie in my arms or in his rocking chair, happily watching the world go by. He was so lazy he would fall asleep whilst he was feeding.

However like Peter, Martin failed to assist with the night feeds! I was just grateful that this time, I was experiencing normal, 'new-mum' tiredness, rather than the indescribable exhaustion I had suffered the first time around!

I enjoyed getting Alex wrapped up and wheeling him out in the early spring sunshine each afternoon to collect Tom from school. Other mothers, rather than sidelining me, as they always had done because of Tom's reputation, would approach me to chat about Alex or to coo over him as he slept, all snug, in his pram. This new-found friendliness cheered me and it was wonderful to feel included in playground conversation rather than be on the edge of it, or indeed the subject of it.

The initial connection I felt had been forged between Tom and Alex did not progress. I tried to involve Tom in caring for his little brother but he was not interested. I would ask him to entertain him whilst I prepared dinner but he could not be bothered. When we were out, he recoiled from pushing the pram. He seemed indifferent to Alex; as though he was invisible. I fretted and worried as Tom spent increasing amounts of time in his room. Attempts to coax him out proved futile; he seemed to prefer doing his own thing.

At least his behaviour had improved and we were going through a quieter, calmer phase. Complaints from school had eased. I stopped keeping behaviour diaries. There were less incidents taking place whilst he was at his dad's. It was definitely as though the birth of Alex could have altered him in some way.

I guess that for a while, I took my eye off the ball. However it bounced back at full pelt and smacked me hard, squarely in the face.

Holiday Memories

September 2002 (8 years, 9 months)

Soon after, we attempted a week away at the coast. The journey was horrendous!

Tom travelled in the middle as he had damaged the seatbelt behind Martin. But he kept unclipping himself and trying to clamber into the front of the car. Or he would boot us through the backs of the seats. Then without warning he threw up! As we set off again Alex suddenly began shrieking, so we pulled back over.

"Tom, Tom!" was all that was audible between sobs. As I shifted the hand that clutched his back; there was a huge purply patch which appeared to have been nipped and twisted. Other marks on his back indicated that he might have been repeatedly poked.

"You nasty little bully!" Martin's gaze travelled from Alex's back into Tom's defiant eyes.

"How could you do that to your little brother?" I added, gathering Alex in my arms to comfort him. I was going to have to step up my vigilance.

When we finally arrived, we decided to go out for a pub lunch. Tom vanished into the toilet. After fifteen minutes I sent Martin to investigate.

"He says he won't be a minute." He retook his place at the table. "It stinks in there! I don't know what he's up to."

"Well his tummy wasn't too good on the journey." Seizing the menu, I began scanning it. "Maybe it's that."

Tom eventually joined us. His shirt sleeves were soaked. I absently observed as a man went into the toilets but reappeared straightaway, visibly gagging, before striding over to the bar. A member of staff man then entered the men's toilets. He exited in a similar instant way; horror etched on his face.

"Martin," I hissed, my appetite starting to wane. "Will you go and see what Tom's done in there?

Hesitantly he headed for the toilets but immediately emerged, looking grim-faced.

"Let's get out of here." He gestured towards the door. "I'll tell you in the car. Just go." As we got through the door, he snarled at Tom: "You dirty little git!"

"What on earth has he done?" I slid into the car.

"Smeared poo everywhere." He slammed himself into the driving seat and rested his head onto the steering wheel. "It's all over the walls, floor, even the door."

In hindsight, Tom should have been frogmarched back in there, made him own up and clean it. But I was too ashamed.

Whenever my back was turned that week, Tom delighted in making Alex squeal in pain. By nipping, poking or trying to squash him. The constant vigil I had to keep wore me out! Inevitably the time passed with Martin and I alternating over who took charge of which child. So much for a family holiday!

Once when I took them together at a play area beside a river, I ended up weeping with exasperation. Goodness knows what passers-by must have thought! Tom had eaten his ice cream and was trying to steal Alex's. When reprimanded, he was abusive before storming off. Half an hour elapsed before I discovered him, hiding up a tree in nearby woods.

He wanted *everything!* Sometimes, we indulged him. At other times, if we refused, the tantrums heightened like a hurricane. Swearing at the peak of his voice, he would make it known to anyone within earshot how he never got anything, and then he would punch or kick whatever was available. He was unstoppable. I was at my wits end!

After the 'holiday,' one of my first ports of call was my GP. Again.

"We don't prescribe it *lightly*," she tried to explain when I begged for Ritalin. "It can cause all sorts of other problems, like stunted growth, developmental problems *and* disturbed sleep."

I laughed. "The fact that he is weeing in corners and smearing poo everywhere would illustrate his already apparent developmental problems! *Twice* whilst we were on holiday! I thought my days of having to rid walls of his excrement were well behind me! And *disturbed sleep!*" My voice probably sounded as manic as I felt at that moment! "He doesn't sleep! Never before the early hours. Even when he does drop off, he wakes up over and over again. He's then up at the crack of dawn!"

"I can't prescribe Ritalin," she repeated. "It's such a new drug and I am reluctant to make the existing problems even worse." She pondered for a moment. "How about I refer you to the 0-19 Team again?"

"The 0-19 Team?" I sniffed, feeling all hope fade out of me like air from a puncture.

"If you *really* convey the problems to them, they might be able to refer you onto someone more specialised." She began typing onto her computer.

"Like who?"

"A child psychologist or psychiatrist even."

"And then what?"

"They would perhaps be in a position to make an attempt at a diagnosis, possibly making medication more of an option."

I felt hopeful at this so agreed for the referral to go ahead.

"There's a bit of a waiting list at the moment," she warned. "You might have to wait for a few weeks."

"That's fine. As long as I know something's happening!" I rose to my feet. "It's only now I've had Alex that I see Tom's behaviour in all its severity. It's not right! And if it was something to do with my parenting skills, Alex would be the same, surely!"

"I know. No one's blaming you."

Bullying Incident 1

Finally the appointment with the 0-19 Team dawned. Elizabeth had agreed to accompany me as I was dreading it. As usual, I was convinced I would be criticised and condemned. First, she came to our house for a preparatory cup of tea.

"Just tell it like it is," she advised as we sat watching Alex play with his cars. "And so will I. They *have* to listen this time."

The children sat together at the table for lunch.

"For God's sake, Tom!" Elizabeth glanced at him in disapproval. "Use your cutlery." She pushed his fork closer to him. "Your table manners are getting worse."

He was attempting to eat spaghetti with his fingers. It splattered the floor and table.

"It's like this every mealtime!" I ran a face flannel under the tap. "Isn't he like this when you've got him?"

"Yes, he is," she admitted, catching the flannel I flung to her. "To be honest, we've learnt to avoid stuff like spaghetti!"

My gaze wandered from his sauce-stained face to Alex, carefully spooning spaghetti from his dish to his mouth. At nearly two years old, he had hardly spilled a morsel!

As the time for leaving neared, Elizabeth rinsed the cups whilst I rummaged around for coats and shoes. Then an ear-splitting scream leapt through the door of the living room.

Left momentarily unattended, Tom had seized his opportunity to attack Alex. Springing from the room, he raced past me up the stairs. I ran in to investigate with Elizabeth in hot pursuit. Alex's scream was actually silent. His face was contorted in pain.

"Breathe!" I ordered, shaking him.

As he gasped, the screams started leaving him. As any mother knows, when your child is small they have different sorts of cries for various things. Hunger, tiredness, boredom, pain. This one was awful. Not yet able to talk properly, we could only assume the pain originated from the ear he clutched. Elizabeth gently moved his hand.

"Oh my God!" My eyes travelled to the site of my baby boy's earlobe, blackening with injury.

The 0-19 Team (again)

January 2003 (9 years, 1 month)

"Did you do that to your brother?" The man seemed shocked as he questioned a defiant-looking Tom.

"I gather this is not the first time your doctor's referred you," he asserted, turning to me.

"No, it's the third." I reclined back in the comfortable chair, leaning my arms on the rests. "I hoping we're going to get somewhere this time."

He extracted a form and pen from his briefcase. "Well, I can promise to listen, but what will happen beyond that, I can't say at the moment."

Elizabeth grasped every chance to insert her own opinions and experiences about Tom as the dialogue progressed. After all, she and Peter took charge of him nearly every weekend.

Discussing Tom so negatively in front of him made me feel guilty. However that feeling dissipated each time I glanced at Alex's swollen ear.

I revisited Tom's babyhood; the sleeplessness, breakages, tantrums and soiling: the urinating, outbursts and his bullying of other children.

Alex played in the middle of us all, surrounded by some cars he had discovered. Tom concealed himself behind my chair, eerily quiet as he fiddled with something. At first I didn't notice his activity.

"Tom, what're you doing?" Elizabeth bent down towards him and extracted some scissors.

He had been cutting up his clothes and had 'unpicked' the stitching from one of his shoes. His trouser leg was cut up one side and he had snipped a hole in his jumper. *Surely, the man had to do something!* I thought, triumphantly. He looked lost in contemplation.

"I'm going to refer you to the Child and Adolescent Mental Health Team," he finally announced, writing something on the bottom of his form. "I think we should get Tom assessed by a child psychiatrist." I felt like punching the air in jubilation. *At last!*

As we let ourselves out of the building, I knew I should be meting out sanctions for the behaviour Tom had displayed that day, but a gnawing little voice sounded within me. *All this is not his fault. He did not choose to be like this. There is something wrong with him.* And it was starting to seem as though we may get it sorted out!

More Humiliation

September 2003 (9 years, 9 months)

Tom had reached the statutory age for sex education. As a result, his pictures became more graphic and suggestive. I worried myself sick about him. My fears were evidently well-founded when my friend Joanne telephoned me one afternoon following our visit to her house.

"Sarah, I'm telling you this because you need to know," she began.

"What's happened?" *Aaargh, what now!" I screamed inwardly.*

"It's Tom."

"What's he done?" I nestled the phone in the crook of my neck as I poured drinks for the kids.

"Well," she hesitated. "Firstly he asked Rebecca to show him her knickers and then said he would give her chocolate if she sucked his willy. It happened while they were in the garden."

"Whaaaat!" I splashed juice everywhere. Her little girl was only six.

"I won't say anything to Paul," she affirmed, referring to her partner. "And I've told Rebecca not to either. He would have a real go at you."

"I know." Tears were seeping down my cheeks as I sank onto a dining chair. "Tom's on the waiting list to see a child psychiatrist. Hopefully I'll start getting help with him soon, you know about the problems I've always had with......."

"Of course I know." "I'm not blaming you. I just hope to God that eventually one of these so-called specialists gives him, and you, some support. I've no idea how you've coped all this time."

*

Once we allowed him a friend to stay overnight. Once was enough.

Just after two in the morning, Tom swore at me when I ordered them to be quiet. When I returned a short time later, he hurled a book at me! Finally I sent Martin in and he sent Tom's exhausted-looking friend to sleep on the sofa.

"You shouldn't speak to your mum like that." I overheard him hiss at Tom once or twice the next morning.

"When can I go home?" he kept asking as we waited for his mum to collect him. That was the last time he and Tom played.

It was a similar story with all the children he encountered. Upon meeting a potential friend, he would monopolise and try to control them. Inevitably, he would lash out if they tried to exert their own personalities. So he continued to live as a bit of a loner.

Sometimes, I felt my heart would break for him. But I felt optimistic that all this would improve once I had persuaded the powers that be that he needed Ritalin.

I was at a complete loss of what to do. In my teacher training at university, I had been reading about using *positive behaviour strategies*. This meant ignoring anything negative as much as possible and rewarding his positive aspects, however marginalised! I leapt upon episodes of him behaving calmly and praise him to the skies.

I made endless promises of rewards. *If the teacher doesn't speak to me at the end of the school day, we'll spend an hour at the park. If you get through the week without being in trouble at school, you can go bowling. If you settle down and go to sleep, I'll take you swimming tomorrow, etc, etc.*

Maybe I was just setting him up to fail though because he did not possess the concentration to retain what I had promised and would, before long, be unable to fulfil the criterion necessary to gain the reward. There would then be hell to pay. Never would he forget a half-promise and would pursue me relentlessly. Screaming at me; he would lash out at all around him and stamp his feet in fury.

On occasion he turned the anger inwards and would beat himself in his face or head with his fists. It was horrifying to witness. On several occasions, I attempted to bring forward the appointment to see the child psychiatrist. But, we had to wait until we made it to the top of the waiting list.

Tom's Teacher

October 2003 (9 years, 10 months)

    A stern, male teacher may have had a handle on him. So my heart plunged when I met his next teacher. She seemed young and barely stood taller than Tom. Perhaps I was mistaken to judge her on appearance but I could not help worrying that he would make mincemeat of her!
    Two weeks into the half-term, she admitted she could not manage. I listened sympathetically as she recounted various episodes she had endured in her brief time as his teacher.
    "It doesn't matter what warnings I give; he just laughs at me."
    "The whole class is disrupted. They don't agree with what he's doing, but they all stop to laugh at him. This just eggs him on even more!"
    "His language is foul. Every colleague I've have spoken to, can't believe that he's still in mainstream school."
    "He bullies, he destroys things."
    "There's no point in me trying to teach him if I can't even get him to behave himself."
    "My teaching assistant is refusing to work with him. She can't manage him either."
    As we talked in the empty classroom, she seemed near to tears. I felt wretched and tried letting her know that I had been having awful trouble with him since his birth, and that she was just one in a long queue of his *victims!*

The Head Teacher

"I always suspected we'd get to this point," asserted Mrs Armstrong, peering at me from behind her desk as though I might have a solution stashed down my sock.

"I have told you we're on the list to see a child psychiatrist, haven't I?"

"Yes, several times!" She nodded, wearily.

"I'm sure once he is diagnosed with ADHD, he will be prescribed Ritalin, then he will sleep better, calm down and his behaviour will improve and...."

"But that doesn't solve the immediate problem." Standing up, she wandered around to the front of her desk and perched herself on the edge of it. "What do we do about him in the meantime?"

His teacher, Miss Thomson dropped her forehead onto her hand. "I can't go on teaching him. Not like he is. My class is out of control with him amongst it. I'm beginning to question whether I'm even cut out for teaching!" Her voice wobbled around the cluttered interior of the headmistresses' office.

"What if we get help for him?" Mrs Armstrong spoke again, resting her arm on that of Miss Thomson's.

"I've been trying to get help for years!" *Why now?*

"He'd meet the criteria for funding now," Mrs Armstrong insisted, looking thoughtful. "We'd have more hope of it being granted just for five *half* days. We're unlikely to get full days. Would you say he's worse in the morning or afternoon?" She leaned over me to extract a file from her bookshelf.

Miss Thomson pondered for a moment. "Afternoons probably. We always do maths and English in the morning and the class are calmer generally. Afternoons tend to be less structured, meaning he's more likely to go off the rails."

"That's settled then. I'll apply for funding for afternoons." announced Mrs Armstrong, sliding a sheet of paper from a plastic sleeve within her file.

I watched her, confused. "What does that mean?"

"It's not easy to get awarded," she explained, scanning down the form. "Normally children have to exhibit severe learning difficulties. But it we're successful it means we could use a one-to-one learning mentor for him. Someone to help with his work, give him frequent behaviour reminders and hopefully keep him on task." She glanced towards Miss Thomson, who appeared to have cheered slightly. "Then if he gets too much, the mentor would be able to remove him from the classroom situation to let off steam until he calms down."

"That sounds promising." I began to feel brighter too. "Do you think it will be granted?" We definitely seemed to be running out of other options.

"I believe we've got a strong case. It could well make the difference between him making it through this school or having to attend a more specialised school."

The Educational Psychologist

Within two weeks I attended an early morning meeting with a fierce looking man who was going to pronounce judgement on my son after observing him over the course of an English lesson.

I have included his report here:

SCHOOL ACTION PLUS
EDUCATIONAL PSYCHOLOGIST'S
ASSESSMENT SUMMARY

Basis for this report:
1. Initial discussion with school
2. Meeting with parents and step parents
3. Observation of, and interview with Tom
4. Records of behaviour made at school by staff, and school reports

Background Information and current concerns from Parents and Step Parents

Mum has been concerned since Tom was a baby: hyperactive behaviour and not sleeping at night. At the age of eighteen months, Mum sought help from the 0-19 team through the GP. Although parents concerns are severe, querying ADHD and wanting statementing, Tom can sit as though butter wouldn't melt in his mouth. Mum is now seeking re-referral. Tom's natural parents have separated; Tom lives with his Mum and spends some of the weekend at Dad's house. He used to be better behaved for his Dad, but is now also cheeky and abusive to him.

Behaviours causing concern more recently have included:
- Extensive breakages: he has smashed everything Mum has owned (TV, video, ornaments as well as his own toys.) He also recently in temper broke a window.
- The problem with sleeping, which is getting worse. At home Tom won't keep still; he sits upside down on the settee and talks constantly.

- Aggression towards his younger brother, Alex, whom Mum can't leave alone in the same room as Tom: he is jealous and has bullied/bruised him and put his hands around his throat. He lashes out at his Step Mum who has had to restrain him from hurting her.
- Wetting and soiling: although Tom is toilet trained, he wees in corners of his bedroom and recently smeared faeces in the toilets on holiday. He admitted this to me saying *I did it because I don't like myself.*
- Tom is lonely and unhappy at school. He says he hasn't any friends, that nobody likes him and that it is boring; he doesn't want to go. He says he is *different* and gets upset. Although he is intelligent he can't concentrate and so can't do the work. Parents are worried about high school transition, fearing he will truant.
- Endangering himself and getting into trouble when he plays out: climbing on garage roofs, falling out and starting fights with older children. Other parents complain about him. Tom's parents are embarrassed to take him anywhere in public. More and more they have had to try and isolate him and not let him play out. In the summer holidays (03), on a caravan park, he was terrible, not going to sleep until 2am, demanding money and having tantrums in public.
- They fear he is going to cause himself injury – he sneaks knives into his bedroom, he jumps off roofs and he head bangs/hurts himself.
- He is clumsy/not well co-ordinated, struggles to use a knife and fork and is unable to tie his shoelaces.

At home parents run behaviour programmes with charts and Tom is interested in the idea of having goals to work towards. But if he doesn't earn his reward, he steals it.

Background from School Staff

Tom was difficult to manage in reception class, for example pulling down his own and others' pants; and he had a difficult year in year 2. He calmed down a little in year 3 with a male teacher. But from the Christmas in year 4 (with another male teacher) he deteriorated again. Tom has acquired a name for himself and tends to get blamed by his class even when an incident is not his fault. In school he can be reasoned with; he responds well to 1:1 support. But there are still regular incidents causing concern:

Aggression towards his peers, threatening aggression, and making hurtful remarks; answering back and shouting at staff, angrily banging doors/furniture; in July he blocked the toilets with toilet rolls. School have maintained diary records of his incidents so they are not listed more fully here.

In interview and observation in class

A morning lesson I observed in his Year 5 class began calmly. Tom started as he was expected to do with quiet reading, joined in the class prayers appropriately, and raised his hand when he wanted the teacher's attention. It took him longer to settle to a writing task than it had to settle to reading, asking for books/equipment, taking a child's pencil from another table then denying it, talking and singing instead of writing, obviously looking for others attention/approval. At the end of the writing period he threw his book across the table onto the floor, but picked it up without comment when told to do so. He frequently frowned. During an overhead projector presentation of a poem, by the teacher, he was restless in his chair, and yawning, rocking back, slouching down, lifting the group's table up and down with his knees, etc. However he answered questions well (e.g. suggesting rhyming words for a poem and defining what adjectives were) and when it was his turn to read aloud to the class, he read well. The work was clearly within his ability.

I understand that Tom manages better in more structured/ formal morning teaching sessions, but finds afternoon sessions (which I did not see) more difficult.

In 1:1 interview Tom told me that he liked his current teacher and preferred literacy to maths. However year 3 was his best year as they had a number of good school trips. He was reticent in talking about things that went wrong in school or at home but stated there were good and bad moments. He names several friends for me, and staff he liked. Sometimes there were arguments with his friends. Sometimes he was good with his temper; sometimes he couldn't control his anger. He had achieved a certificate the week before I saw him for not fighting and getting into trouble all week.

He felt his behaviour at home and school was about the same. He thought the arrangement of living with Mum and seeing Dad at weekends worked fine, although he felt he got on better with Dad, as there were sometimes arguments with his Mum.

Identified needs

Tom's history suggests a high level of emotional need. This well may be linked with an attachment disorder,** but this diagnosis would be better coming from the Child and Adolescent Mental Health Team. Tom's behaviour has a major impact on his family/families at home. In school he is more unsettled in less structured situations.

Recommendations

To provide increased supervision in afternoons and social times and opportunities to work in 1:1 and small group settings on feelings and anger management, I would support schools' request for 'F Band' funding for inclusion.

Educational Psychologist 24.11.2003

This report is based on one hour of observing Tom.
*** Attachment Disorder is most common in fostered and adopted children but is found in other so-called "normal" families as well - due to divorce, illness or separations. It happens when a child is not properly nurtured in the first few months and years of life. The child, left to cry in hunger, pain or need for cuddling, learns that adults will not help him or her. (Source: Behaviour for Learning)*

The Learning Mentor

To my disappointment it was a lady, nice enough, a little *too* nice in fact! I had fervently hoped a male might have been appointed; someone Tom would be wary of! However, for several weeks, Miss Thomson's complaints quietened down. Tom was given frequent breaks, distracting activities and opportunities to let off steam in the playground. For a while it worked and I began to relax.

But before long, he had gleaned the learning mentor's fallible traits and which buttons to press. She was battling with him. It was not long before I was summoned into school for yet another meeting.

The Chair of Governors

November 2003 (9 years, 11 months)

"I'm Mr Phillips," he announced, gesturing to a seat in front of the desk. "The Chair of Governors."

"Oh, erm, nice to meet you." I surveyed him expectantly. *Was it?*

"I'd like to discuss Tom." Pausing, he shuffled through a file before him. "As you're aware, this school has persevered against all his problems."

"I know, and I'm grateful." I leaned forward in my chair.

"The thing is; we're reaching the end of the line." Halting his paper shuffling, he linked his hands together on the large mahogany desk belonging to Mrs Armstrong. "Complaints from other parents are mounting and the next school year is important. We've SATS to consider, not to mention the transition to high school."

"Yes." *Oh God, what was he saying to me?*

"We *have* to consider the needs and welfare of *all* out pupils in school, not just Tom." His gaze was boring into me.

"I know." I felt childlike and defenceless against this big, important man who seemed to be finally writing off my son.

"This meeting is the first step towards Tom being permanently excluded from this school." His voice had become sterner. "It is a verbal warning that his behaviour *has* to improve, most considerably, with immediate effect."

"But what if it doesn't? ...." I sat bolt upright in my chair, my heart doing somersaults. *Surely he wasn't going to end up expelled! Not from primary school!* "I'll try talking to him obviously but I've tried everything already and........"

"The next step will be a written warning." His face displayed scant emotion. "After that if there is still no improvement, I'm afraid you will receive a letter informing you to withdraw him from this school."

"But then what would I do?"

"You could apply for a place at other mainstream schools in the area – if they have places available. I have to warn you though, that other schools would be reluctant to accept him if he'd been excluded from here. You might be looking at a pupil referral unit."

"What's that?" I felt deflated and small as I perched before him.

"A secure unit where staff are specifically trained to deal with severe problem behaviours; there are appropriate facilities and smaller class sizes." By his tone of voice, I could tell that he deemed it an appropriate environment for Tom.

"But surely he would only get worse if forced to spend his days with other like-minded children?"

He shrugged. Like he had indicated, his priority was the rest of the children. It was abundantly clear to me that the school wanted Tom out. They'd had enough.

The Child Psychiatrist

Eventually, hope arrived in the form of an appointment. All of us, including Elizabeth, Peter and even Tom, had to fill an array of questionnaires regarding relationships, concentration, sleep and so on.

I helped Tom with his. One question was *do you have enjoyable time with your friends?* The responses to choose from were *often, sometimes, rarely* and *never.* After ticking *never*, he turned to me.

"No one wants to play with me cos I'm bad." His blue eyes emitted a sadness that sliced straight into my heart.

"You're not bad, you daft thing!" I tried to hug him. His body went rigid and I could sense him squirming. He had *never* done hugs.

"Right Tom." We were hunched together at the kitchen table. "What answer shall we give for this question? *Do you feel you have someone you can talk to?*"

Again he answered *never.*

"But you know you can always talk to me." My voice echoed around the kitchen competing for airspace with the din of the washer's spin cycle. "Or Martin, or your dad and Elizabeth."

Shrugging with indifference, he began scanning the next question. It delighted me that he managed to concentrate for several minutes as his form was completed. Surely it was a positive omen about the impending appointment? I felt certain help was imminent.

The four adults in his life had to attend the first meeting without Tom. We waited nervously in a shiny clinical room, squinting at each other as the sharp sunlight bounced off the gleaming white walls. The only reassuring touches in this stark room were a box of tissues and a basket of pot pourri. Feeling jittery, I leaned forward to inhale its scent. It was lavender-ish, but an improvement on the surrounding 'dettolly' smell.

Peter shot me a peculiar look. "I don't know what you expect to achieve by this Sarah." Elizabeth glowered at him. "Why should this person be any different from the others?"

"Look, it's worth a try. Just back me up, will you."

A demure, dark-haired woman entered the room.

"I'm Victoria Harris." She closed the door with great care as though she was trying not to disturb something. "Nice to meet you all." As she shook each of our hands, we introduced ourselves. She was quietly spoken and her voice had a 'posh' edge. Although expensively dressed, she looked young, perhaps a recent graduate, my first impression was certainly negative enough to make me feel dubious as to whether she would be able to help.

"Right first I need to get some background." She nodded towards me. "I'll begin with you Sarah." This caused me to feel mildly defensive. "Family, medical history, that sort of thing. For a moment I tussled with the notion of omitting the fact that I had been in care in my teens. Then I decided not to. *What would be the point?* In any case, she hardly flinched when I mentioned it. Apparently, she was not of the *'abused parents become abusers'* brigade. Then the questions were directed to the others whilst she frantically scribbled notes on her pad.

"I'm sure you're tired of going over it all over and over again, but we do need to go right back to the beginning and work forwards." I felt reassured by her apparent efficiency. "To put a clear picture together I have to learn *everything*."

"How long's this appointment?" I joked, starting to relax a little.

She smiled. Don't worry; we'll get through what we can." Extracting her diary from her bag, she began leafing through it as she spoke. "At the next appointment, I'd like to meet Tom as well, so I can observe his behaviour and interaction with all of you.

Her questioning probed my pregnancy and the birth, my early days with Tom and his sleeping patterns. *Had he been a planned baby? Was I well after birth? Any depression? What support had I had? How did he sleep? How did we bond?*

There was no point in being anything other than honest. Support from anyone had been in short supply back then. It had been a struggle, but we had got by. Tom was my only child then; I had not worked for the first eighteen months so he was my entire life; we were inseparable. It had not been until he was approaching two, that I had been forced to accept there was something not right and had sought support. It had been painful for me to admit there was a problem with my own child but it was something that I would have always had to face up to eventually.

Not all the questions were directed at me, which I was pleased about. Everybody else was included in the discussion. Her thoroughness gave me confidence and I was disappointed when the ninety minute appointment came to an abrupt close.

The Follow-up Appointment

January 2004 (10 years, 1 month)

The subsequent meeting included Tom. There was an air of expectation as we convened. Tom shifted uncomfortably in his seat, avoiding Victoria's eye as he fiddled with everything.

"Have you got a car?" he enquired, when she questioned him about how he was progressing at school. His gaze wandered about the room; he was evidently having trouble concentrating on her questions.

"I've heard you've a talent for drawing." She offered him paper and pencils. Perhaps you could draw whilst we talk."

As he sketched, Sarah continued to try and hold his attention. His answers were given as a shrug or in one word. Not once did he smile, but he seemed calm. Part of me wanted him to display his destructive behaviour, if only to quantify our claims!

True to form though, he drew one of his violent shooting pictures.

"Can you tell me about your picture?" Sarah got up and studied it over his shoulder, without portraying any other reaction.

"He's the baddie, he's the baddie as well and he's just shot him in the head."

"Oh." She slouched back down. "What other pictures can you draw?"

"I can't be bothered!" He slung the paper and pencil onto the floor.

"Tom, pick them up."

"No, you pick them up." He flung his body as far back in the seat as it would go.

"You threw it down." Peter frowned towards him.

Elizabeth bent down and retrieved the items from the floor.

Tom jumped up, throwing his chair back with a scrape that made me shiver, and then tried to vacate the room.

"Get back here now!" I ordered, secretly glad that he was playing up!

"Get lost." The door slammed behind him with Victoria in pursuit. The four of us stared at each other. Words were not exchanged.

Hallelujah! I am finally being listened to!

Getting Somewhere

May 2004 (10 years, 5 months)

Week after week we attended. Sometimes with Tom; sometimes without. The four of us would go, or just Martin and I, or Peter and Elizabeth. Tom, as he became more familiar with Victoria and the stifling consulting room, was starting to let his guard slip and display more 'Tom-like' behaviour!

Eventually Victoria announced that she was in a position to make a vague diagnosis. I shifted in my seat. *ADHD, Ritalin.....please!*

"Although traits of his behaviour are consistent with ADHD, I don't believe that is the underlying problem."
"So you don't think it's ADHD?" Leaning forward, I felt disappointed that she disagreed with me.
"No."
"But he's got *every* symptom of it in abundance. I've been with him every single day of
his life and know him better than *anyone*."
"I'm not disputing your opinion," she insisted gently. "Just that his symptoms point more to a conduct disorder."
"Conduct disorder," I echoed. Finally, a name! A condition! Something! Anything! But what did it mean?
"It's an 'umbrella' term," she explained, shaping her hands in the air like an umbrella. "It embodies all sorts of different problems and behaviours that Tom is exhibiting.
"Is it treatable?" "I'm afraid not, however it can be managed."
"How?" I was happy to clutch at the fragments of hope she was offering.

Over subsequent weeks, we considered all sorts of scenarios and methods of dealing with them. In her calm manner, she helped me (and the others to a lesser extent) realise that Tom was, well Tom. A magic wand was not available to alter him.

But we could change ourselves hence, I became forced to analyse my reactions to his behaviour. Nagging, exasperated, shouting responses and the alternatives to them such as giving a warning, then a sanction, and then following things through. Calmly and quietly.

I was the adult, he the child. If I stayed composed then I may have some hope of keeping him calm. This of course applied to his other carers.

Victoria advocated the importance of my doing an activity alone, just with Tom, without Alex or Martin there for a minimum of one hour each week. Something of *his* choosing, so he would feel he had me all to himself. I nodded, knowing this was worth a try. From having had me to himself for eight years, he now had to 'share' me with Alex. It was something I had not considered before.

We discussed boundaries, consequences and distractions. All of this went over several appointments. But ultimately I felt empowered and more in control. Suddenly I had a better understanding of what I was dealing with.

I was going to give it everything I had to get his behaviour straightened out. Every scrap of advice Victoria had offered would be implemented, particularly the firming up of boundaries and being vigilant over additives in his diet.

A fresh start would be the way forward; a brand new school and a more tolerant mother. There was no way I was ever going to give up on him!

Conduct Disorder

Conduct Disorder (CD) is a disruptive type of behavioural disorder in which a child routinely violates the personal rights of others and shows no care for others' property. CD is more diagnosed in boys than girls and affects approximately five percent of the population under 15 years of age in the United Kingdom.

Signs/Symptoms of Conduct Disorder

There are a variety of signs/symptoms of conduct disorder, though for a formal diagnosis there must be at least one shown and it must be shown for a period of more than six months. Common signs/symptoms of CD include aggressive behaviours toward others or animals, destructive behaviours towards the property of others including harming or destroying items (including cars and homes), lying to others, stealing from others and playing truant from school. Older children and teens may also engage in behaviours harmful to themselves such as smoking and tobacco use, alcohol use, substance abuse and engaging in unprotected sexual activities.

Diagnosing Conduct Disorder

A diagnosis of Conduct Disorder must be made by a professional in child psychology. There are two types of conduct disorder and the distinction is marked by age. Child-Onset Type CD is diagnosed when at least one sign or symptom is shown, for at least six months, prior to the age of 10 years. Adolescent-Onset Type CD is diagnosed when at least one sign or symptom is show, for at least six months, after the age of 10 years but no signs or symptoms were shown prior to the age of 10 years. CD may also be described as mild, moderate or severe. Children with mild CD will exhibit few signs/symptoms and cause little harm to others. Children with moderate CD will exhibit multiple signs/symptoms and cause harm to others. Children with severe

CD will exhibit signs/symptoms and will cause much harm to others through their actions or the consequences of their actions.

Treating Conduct Disorder

The method of treatment selected for a child with Conduct Disorder will be determined by the child's age, signs/symptoms, and tolerance for or comfort with medications and/or therapies. Main approaches to treatment include cognitive-behavioural therapy which helps to improve a child's problem-solving, communication, impulse control and anger management skills, family therapy/counselling and possibly medication to treat the signs/symptoms of CD.

Living with Conduct Disorder

It is imperative that a child diagnosed with Conduct Disorder has a supportive family and home environment. Not only is this important for following whatever treatment programme is devised, but it helps the child realise that they are still loved and appreciated despite their behaviours. A healthy diet and plenty of exercise is also essential for children being treated for CD. Notifying teachers and tutors of a diagnosis of CD is also significant as it will help the child feel supported at school and notify educators of the child's special needs.

Conduct Disorder is a behavioural disorder characterised by aggression, defiance and antisocial behaviour. CD must be diagnosed by a child psychology expert, and treatment may include cognitive-behavioural therapy, family counselling and/or medication to treat the signs/symptoms of the disorder. Families living with CD should remain supportive and loving towards the child with the disorder, and notify teachers and tutors so that the child will be supported at school as well.

Source: www.kidsbehaviour.co.uk › Behavioural Disorders

Another Bullying Incident

November 2004 (10 years, 11 months)

It became apparent as Alex approached three-years-old, that he had asthma. Luckily, Elizabeth and Peter lived close by and would collect Tom at short notice, enabling me to get Alex to hospital. His condition would deteriorate quickly if he was not given steroids and a nebuliser. Twice he ended up in recsus. For me, as his mother, it was terrifying and I subsequently became neurotic with ensuring his room was dust-free, and safeguarding him from traffic fumes and cigarette smoke. Tom resented the attention I was 'lavishing' on him.

"I love you both the same," I would repeatedly assure him, when he whinged that I only cared about Alex.

"I don't see why you have to *sleep* at hospital with him," he pouted. "It's not like he'd care if you went home." I had left Alex with Martin at the hospital, in order to return home for some things, then to drop Tom off with Elizabeth and Peter.

"Tom, if you were ill or hurt in hospital, I'd stay with you too," I draped my arm around his shoulder. "Hopefully it's just for a night or two."

"I hate you!" He yanked himself from my embrace and stormed through the front door towards the car. "And I hate *him* even more!"

Sadly, he seemed to mean it. Worryingly, he often emptied Alex's asthma inhalers by repeatedly pressing them. Alex's medication was being trialled and his asthma was out of control. I ordered extra inhalers and hid them everywhere.

His fifth asthma attack, when he was nearly four-years-old was by far the most severe one. Our hospital stay lasted five endless days.

"We're going to try him on Seretide," stated the consultant before he discharged him. "It's not normally given to children under twelve but Alex is a big lad for his age. I think he'll tolerate it. It's been successful; it's a preventer *and* reliever in one."

On leaving the hospital I went directly to collect Tom, promising to treat him to a takeaway supper and a DVD. Alex seemed worn out so I decided to give him an early night, promising Tom that I would be back downstairs soon to watch the film with him.

It was a chilly November night so I helped Alex into his fleecy pyjamas, ensuring he had a vest underneath. Giving him a blast of his new inhaler, I turned back his bedclothes so he could climb in.

"Mummy, it's wet!" Springing straight back out of his bed, he shivered.

"It can't be." But as I smoothed my hand along his sheet, I realised it was sodden with freezing cold water. The bedroom heater had been switched off and his window opened as far as it would go. Yet the curtains had drawn back across to conceal the open window. I called Martin upstairs.

"This is serious!" Martin was grim faced as he ran his hand over Alex's sheet. "Thank God you realised." He shook his head. "If Alex had fallen asleep downstairs, we'd have carried him up and put him in bed in the dark without realising."

"He'd have had icy air wafting on him all night too," I added, pointing to the gaping window.

"He only got out of hospital a few hours ago," Martin went on. "You do realise this is Tom trying to hurt him."

"It's probably my fault too Martin." I hung my head as I scooped Alex into my arms. "I've been wrapped up looking after Alex that I haven't been giving Tom enough attention."

"Don't be ridiculous, Alex is only four!" He pointed angrily towards where Alex was snuggled into my chest. "He's been in bloody hospital! What did Tom expect you to do?"

"He's still a kid himself though!" I nestled my nose into Alex's hair, breathing in his innocent scent.

"And a bloody nasty one at that!" He leaned out of the bedroom door. "Tom get up these stairs NOW!"

Tom appeared in the doorway.

"Why have you soaked Alex's bed?" Martin stood, hands on hips, glaring at Tom.

"I spilt summat, so what."

Playing with Fire 1

One morning I was baffled to wake at seven-thirty to a silent, still house. Tom was usually awake from about six o'clock. I tiptoed up to his room. Pushing his door open, I was greeted by the stench of smouldering rubber and a missing square of carpet in the centre of the room. His bed had been shifted from its usual spot and he was busily hacking a similar sized square from the area under his bed with a lethal-looking kitchen knife.

"What do you think you're doing?" I stared in horror at his activity from the doorway.

My voice startled him. "Nowt!"

A box of matches sat on his windowsill with a large square of charred carpet perched beside them. *That's what he was doing!* Replacing burnt carpet with a square from beneath his bed in the hope I wouldn't notice. As my stunned gaze travelled from his windowsill back towards him, I noticed several scorch marks along his wall. He appeared to have held a flame to it. *It was a miracle the house was still standing!*

"You stupid boy!" Marching to the window, I snatched up the matches.

"I was only messing about," he smirked, still maintaining his carpet cutting.

"You could have burnt the bloody house down!" Striding towards him, I thrust my hand out for the knife.

"Take a chill pill Mum." Thankfully he placed the knife in my hand without argument.

"Where did you get the matches?"

"I dunno."

"Right you can stay up here all morning." I swiped at the piece of carpet he had chopped out. "I can't believe you could be so idiotic!"

In addition to the scorch damage, there was litter everywhere, the familiar stench of urine and a stereo that lay in bits.

"Are you going to give me some breakfast or are you going to STARVE me? I hate you, you stupid COW!"

Tinsel and Tantrums

December 2004 (nearly 11 years)

Before we knew it, Christmas was upon us. Tom was up at around five and immediately went to wake Alex. Exasperated, I knew any possibility of sleep had vanished. I tiptoed downstairs in the darkness with them.

"Has he been?" I nudged an excited Alex as we neared the foot of the stairs.

"There's no such thing as....."

"Ssssh," I scolded Tom. "Don't spoil it for him."

Alex gasped when he noticed that Santa had drunk his glass of Baileys and saw that only a crumb remained of the mince pie.

"Look Mummy," he exclaimed, reaching for the stump of carrot that Rudolf had left.

"You're dumb," Tom jeered, bursting into the living room.

They both gasped as they surveyed the presents beneath the tree. Tom skidded across the carpet and began tearing into them.

"No, that pile's yours," I redirected Tom to the other mound beside the tree.

"But that's smaller," he wailed, making mental comparisons. "That's not fair. He's got more presents than me!"

"You've both had exactly the same spent on you," I sighed.

"But he's got more. *Why* has he got more?"

"Oh for God's sake Tom. The stuff you've got is more expensive. Stop being ridiculous."

Within several minutes, Tom had ripped his presents open.

"Oh." He unearthed a parcel containing new clothes. Then *"what have you bought me books for?"* Then *"crap"* as he opened a game for his console from my sister.

He was delighted however, with his portable DVD player.

"How much did it cost?" he demanded, waving in the air.

"Tom, don't ask how much things cost. It's rude."

"Is that it?" He rummaged amongst the discarded wrapping paper. "Is that all I get?"

I felt deflated, having struggled for two months to ensure adequate presents for my boys. They had been carefully planned and like lots of parents, had left me short of money, with only enough left aside to ensure Tom had an enjoyable 11th birthday which was a week away.

The portable DVD player unfortunately did not last long. In a rage over something, Tom slammed it shut, irreparably damaging its fragile screen. I wanted to weep at the wasted money, but what really affected me, was the fact that he had robbed himself of his main Christmas present. When I refused to replace it, he vented his temper elsewhere in his bedroom. He tore down his curtains and broke the glass in his window by launching his handheld games console towards it. This now lay in pieces on the carpet. It was one of his most long-standing possessions, having survived an entire year before meeting its demise.

For anyone with a destructive child, I would heartily recommend the durable 'Gameboy' console. But even that was not ultimately Tom-proof!

So there it was, Christmas 2004. Tinsel and tantrums. Trying to pacify an impossible child!

His Last Year at Primary School

Tom passed his final primary school year at a different school in the hope that he might reach high school without being permanently excluded. Within my bones, I honestly felt he would mature away from various traits he had been exhibiting. It was just a matter of me keeping a firm rein on him and continuing to persevere. I had faith that everything would ultimately work out!

When we visited the new school, my insides were rattling with anxiety. I had given him a pep talk (well, read the riot act), but he had been promised a treat if he managed a tour of the school without causing any kind of scene!

It was closer to our home and miraculously the school agreed a space for him with an immediate start. They would send for his old school records in due course. I had to complete several forms but found myself skirting around the 'further information' section.

History of Conduct Disorder. I wrote in small writing. *Currently under specialist and making improvement. Please telephone if you require any more information.*

It was not long before his new teacher did. When I had been introduced to him on Tom's first day, I had been delighted. An older teacher, he probably approaching retirement, but he seemed strict. He lurked behind a beard, filling me with belief that Tom would unable to master him!

Six weeks elapsed before I received the call.

"This is Mr Brown." He even *sounded* a bit forbidding!

"Has Tom settled in OK?" I stammered.

"A little *too* well, I'm afraid! He drew a slow breath. "Thomas has joined this school at a late stage in his primary career and one would expect such a child to be, how we shall put it, a tad reserved in his dealings with new teachers and other pupils."

"But?"

"We appear to be wrestling for one-upmanship. Evidently, he is an intelligent boy but seems to be challenging that intelligence into activities that have little to do with school work. In other words, he's causing mayhem and I *won't* tolerate it!"

"I agree with you." Suddenly, I felt guilty for not giving him prior warning. But maybe if I had, an immediate opinion would have been formed of Tom without giving him a chance to settle in first.

"Do we have your blessing to deal with Tom as we see fit?"

"Of course! But what do you mean?" *Do what you want!*

"Segregation, detentions; lunchtime and after school." He paused and breathed deeply again. "Doing work whilst others are enjoying art, missing the school trip, being banned from the school disco, being left out of cycle training; in other words, all the things that I know will get to him."

"Yes, do all that, you have my complete blessing! I'm surprised you needed to ask! And if there's anything I can do to support you, just let me know."

"Just don't be upset if he comes home moaning about me! My bark is worse than my bite!"

I laughed, relieved I had moved him. For the rest of the school year, Tom miraculously was in hand at school.

After School Club

February 2005 (11 years, 2 months)

Sadly it was a different tale at the after-school club; linked to the school; where I paid for him to be supervised when I had late finishes at university. It was run by several young mums.

Tom soon made his presence felt, meaning that week-after-week I was dragged into office to hear endless accounts of his behaviour. Most of it was the bullying of other children or cheek to staff members. It was low-level stuff at first, but the staff were already becoming frustrated.

"He's the only year six child we have in the club," remarked the officer-in-charge one afternoon after she had hauled me into the office. "All the other children of working parents go home on their own."

"You don't understand," I pleaded. "He'd burn my house down! There's no way he could be trusted!"

"Well you need to have a strong word with him. Because if things don't improve dramatically; we're going to have to ask you to make alternative arrangements."

"I understand; I'll speak to him. I'm sorry you need to keep speaking to me about him. I need this school club place. It just wouldn't be safe for him to go home alone, he's not responsible enough!"

They persevered a bit longer but inevitably, his behaviour deteriorated to the point where parents were complaining about his bullying. Things came to a head when he stole money from the handbag of one of the staff.

I didn't try to change the officer-in-charge's mind when she informed me of their decision to ban him from the club. The shame was overwhelming.

The Transition to High School

Despite his protestations, I insisted on accompanying Tom on his first day at what Alex had dubbed *'big, big school'*. He looked grown up and smart in his new uniform. I harboured huge hopes that high school would provide a turning point. The lump in my throat was enormous as I attempted to hug him.

We gave him the first in a long succession of house keys, hoping that a bit of trust and responsibility would be a positive step forward. I bought him neck cords and key rings to keep them safe. By the third key I stipulated they must remain in his coat's zip-up compartment. Or his bag. But in quick succession he lost his coat *and* his bag. Both containing our house keys. Bus passes were lucky to last more than a couple of days before being mislaid. It was unbelievable.

For Christmas that year, we presented him with his first mobile phone. It was amazing to see him grateful for a change and I prayed that it would not meet the same fate as his present from the previous year. But within four weeks he had lost it and vented his frustration by thumping and kicking walls and doors in the house. Then he trashed his bedroom. Aghast, I listened to the commotion, powerless to intervene.

Replacing missing school jumpers was tiresome and costly. Some parents might have taught him a lesson by enabling him to feel the temperature. But it was a harsh winter and I worried what school would make of me if he did not wear adequate jumpers and coats. Within two terms, he had three different school coats. He was costing me a fortune.

However, that first year at high school passed without major incident. I kept a vigil over his school 'planner,' which contained details of homework, punctuality and behaviour. Points were awarded or taken away according to effort, attainment and compliance. Negative comments in the planner resulted in detentions. Tom was not short of these but I never was I telephoned about him, nor dragged into school that year. Not once!

Maybe we had finally turned a corner?

Happy Holiday!

May 2006 (12 years, 5 months)

To attempt another holiday with Tom in tow was barmy, in hindsight! But it had been nearly two years since we had been anywhere.

On arrival at Butlins I gave him £10, informing him that this was the amount of spending money he would receive on each day of the holiday. It lasted approximately ten minutes before being frittered away in the arcades! Immediately, he requested more and thumped the wall upon this being refused. His rage was only thwarted by the approaching security guard!

Throughout our 'break,' Tom's constant demands for entertainment, food and drink were relentless. With a thirst as immense as always, he would gulp his own drink like he had spent the day in a desert and then guzzle down Alex's.

I spent the week being shouted and sworn at, and having vile names slung at me whenever I said 'no' to him. As the week wore on, I questioned why I had ever bothered to organise a pleasant family holiday. It was anything but.

On our penultimate day; Tom announced he was going swimming. It was an amazing pool, one of the main attractions of the holiday park, with water chutes, wave machines and rapids. We arranged to join him there. But within half an hour he reappeared with bloodshot eyes, reeking of chlorine.

"How come you've come back?" I clattered around the chalet, chucking swimming things into a bag. "We were getting ready to come down."

"I'm not going." He flung himself onto the sofa.

"You look like you've already been." I felt his hair. "How come your hair's wet?"

"I dunno." He licked his lips. "I've been sick."

"Sick? Have you?" I felt his forehead. "You were fine this morning."

"I drank loads of pop, had loads of sweets then went on some rides."

"Well you'd better go and have a lie down for a bit." I poured him a drink before passing him the bucket from under the sink.

"I'm not ill." He sprang up. "I'm alright now."

"Well, you might be feeling a bit better but if you've been sick, you certainly can't go swimming."

After some argument, he agreed to stay at the chalet in front of the TV. However, when we arrived at the pool, it had been closed.

"Why have they shut it?" A woman emerged from the building. From her damp hair and flushed cheeks, she had managed to have a swim.

"Some bloody kid who didn't even bother to get himself out of the water." Grimacing, she explained what had happened. "He just stood there and barfed. Dirty little sod! The place is shut for two days now whilst they filter all the water."

Martin and I exchanged glances. I hoped the woman didn't notice the shameful expression upon my face. *Oh Tom!*

Expensive Trainers

June 2006 (12 years, 6 months)

    Tom was becoming extremely 'label-conscious.' The clothes I presented him with clearly did not match up to the expectations of what he felt he deserved.
    "But I need them Mum!" Some £90 trainers were consuming him and he had been whining about them for most of the morning!
    "They're far too expensive." I stacked plates onto the draining board. "But if they're what you want, you'll have to get some of the money together yourself."
    "Yeah and how am I bloody supposed to do that?" Leaning over me, he filled a glass with water.
    "Get a paper round or something." I wiped my hands on a towel. "That's what I had to do at your age."
    "Yeah right," he began stomping out of the kitchen. "I'm really gonna do a stupid paper round."
    "Well if you were to get half of the money together yourself," I called after him in an effort to compromise, "I'd help you with the rest."
    But that was not good enough for him. The argument rumbled on for days, during which time he became increasingly distressed. Undoubtedly his heart was truly set on these trainers and he expected me to pay for them.
    "Either you buy them or I'll smash up the house!" he eventually screamed before barricading himself in the bathroom. I hammered on the door; worried about the damage he was doing as he banged and crashed around.
    Slumping onto the top step of the staircase, I glumly observed the front door that I hoped Martin would suddenly appear through. An odd sensation was prickling at the nape of my neck. Fear.
    Finally Tom emerged, before trying to barge past me. Racing into the bathroom, I then exhaled with relief as I assessed the damage. *Just a couple of squashed shampoo bottles!* That, I could deal with. Their floral scent drifted up my nose and briefly

composed me. But then I swung around and groaned at the three holes he had booted in the door.

My descent down the stairs passed in a blaze of white fury. I found Tom in the kitchen, calmly preparing a sandwich.

"You little……!" Somehow I refrained from throttling him. "We'll be charged for that damage! How can you carry on like this?" His sandwich making paused as he calmly peered at me, his eyes flashing a piercing shiver of hatred. Then grabbing the kettle, he hurled it to its demise at my feet, before slamming out of the house.

It was the evening before he returned home, wearing just one trainer. I tried to ignore him.

"You'll have to buy me them trainers now," he stated, with an air of victory as he pursued me upstairs.*

*Don't worry. We didn't.

Education Welfare

September 2006 (12 years, 9 months)

For the Attention of the Parent or Carer of Thomas Clifford

It has been brought to our attention that the school attendance of the above named has dropped below 75%. Your child usually does not arrive at school at all or else leaves the school premises shortly after registration.

I am aware that this matter has been brought to your attention on several occasions but as it does not appear to have improved, we are left with no alternative other than to issue you with a formal warning.

It is your duty, as someone having parental responsibility, to ensure that your child attends school regularly.* Failure to do this will result in further action being taken against you which could include prosecution or a fixed penalty of £50.

Yours faithfully

Education Welfare Officer

*I was incensed by this letter. Martin or I would drive him to school each day, drop him at the main entrance and ensure he disappeared inside. Short of remaining with him for the remainder of the school day, I am unsure as to what else we could possibly have done.

More Bullying – At school this time

October 2006 (12 years, 10 months)

"We're ringing with regards to an ongoing bullying problem." It was one of Tom's teachers. It had to be serious if he was calling me in the middle of his lunch break.

I paused intently, awaiting further information. Perhaps things were about to slot into place. No wonder his behaviour at home had deteriorated. If he was being bullied at school, that would also explain the truanting. There would be stern words coming their way if that was the case.

"We have a boy in Tom's class with Asperger's Syndrome," he continued. "Unfortunately, this makes Duane an easy target. He has fallen victim to low-level abuse from Tom for several weeks; name calling, snide remarks, that sort of thing."

My heart plummeted, along with the words of defence I had prepared. Tom was not the victim – he was the bully.

"His parents have lodged a formal complaint. Duane doesn't want to come to school anymore. There are witnesses to what's been going on, mainly other class members, who have seen many incidences of Tom's bullying."

"I don't know what to say............," I began, clenching my eyes shut as though I could somehow block out the shame.

"It's getting worse too. Tom has apparently threatened to smack Duane and the poor lad's beside himself with fear. We're going to have to isolate Tom from class for the rest of the week. Do you think you could try to talk to him about why he's treating another person in this way?"

"Of course." My eyes remained closed the conversation concluded. "I'm ashamed of him."

*

"He's a weirdo," was Tom's response when challenged, as he rode beside me in the car. "A freak. A nerd."

"You nasty, cruel boy," I was struggling to concentrate on the road, unable to bear the spite in his face. "Where did all this hate come from? You weren't brought up like this!"

Playing With Fire 2, Exclusion 1

November 2006 (12 years, 11 months)

Tom was unable to behave, even in the school's isolation unit.

"This is Tom's head of year," boomed a male voice down the phone. "Is that his mum?"

"Yes?" I glanced around as life progressed normally throughout the supermarket I was in.

"I've just left him unattended in the unit." His voice wobbled in anger. Or maybe stress. Or both. "Not even for ten minutes."

"And?" Amidst the beeping of checkouts, I dared not hear what Tom had done this time.

"Lucky I came back when I did! I caught him holding a lighter flame up to a pile of folders!" His words were garbled as though he couldn't get them out fast enough. "One or two had already caught fire!"

"I can't believe he would be so stupid!" I was forgetting where I was as several shoppers peered curiously at me. "It's just one thing after another!"

"I managed to extinguish them without the fire alarms being activated, so at least the whole school didn't have to be evacuated." His voice had evened out a little now. "But it's so serious an incident that we'll be placing him on a three-day fixed-term exclusion. The entire school could have been burnt down!"

Bowing my head, I contemplated having him at home for three days. "I understand. Can you set work for him to do at home?"

"Of course. But he needs to be off the school premises as soon as possible. Can you come and collect him?"

By the time I got there he had run off! The woman on reception stared at me as though I was something she had trodden in. She was obviously a member of the *blame the parents* club!

Hastily, I retreated to my car, half-relieved that I could prolong the inevitable confrontation with Tom until later.

When he made it home that evening he was clearly under the influence of something. As he brushed past me, I caught the scent of an unfamiliar smell, chemically, herby.

"He's stoned," Martin stated flatly as Tom headed for the kitchen. "That's cannabis."

"Give over." I shook my head, refusing to consider the possibility. "It can't be."

Martin nodded to where Tom had begun munching his way through a packet of biscuits while he waited for his dinner to reheat in the microwave. "You'll see."

The three days of him being off school were hell. After the first day, I gave up attempting to force him to do the schoolwork they had set; it was hardly worth the abuse!

The relief I felt upon his return to school was immense! However, within days they were back on the phone.

Exclusion 2

"I'm sorry." It was his head of year on the phone. "We're excluding him again. We've had two incidents today."

"Oh great!" *More* time off college. "Now what?"

"He's damaged a computer after being caught looking at inappropriate material on the internet. Upon being challenged he slammed his fist down onto the keypad. It won't even start up now."

"Will I be billed?" I felt drained.

"There's a possibility that the school's insurance will cover it. The repair bill could be hefty so we'll have to let you know on that."

"What's the other thing?" I enquired, slumping onto a bench in the sunshine.

"He's nicked a bag from another pupil. Luckily we've retrieved it from him. Eventually, he led us to where he had hidden it in the school grounds. Several people saw him take it so I think he realised he was cornered."

"Was anything missing?" The college friend who sat beside me, patted me sympathetically on the arm, innately knowing that the situation I was currently discussing would no doubt be centred around Tom.

"No, thankfully. We would have had to involve the police if that had been the case. I have to say though"……, he inhaled deeply; "he is lucky that we haven't informed them. Next time we won't have a choice."

Exclusion 3

April 2007 (13 years, 4 months)

"I'm sorry to be the bearer of bad news but we're going to have to send him home," stated his head of year, without even introducing himself as I answered the phone. Tom hadn't even managed to last until morning break!

"Why?"

"He's been smoking cannabis on school premises, I'm afraid." Mr Wharton sounded more bemused than usual. "Evidently, he's still under the influence."

"I'm unable to collect him for at least an hour." I glanced towards the clock in the college refectory.

"He needs to be off the premises right away. We can't be having drugs flying around!" Pages rustled in the background. "Can we contact his father?"

"Be my guest."

Peter looked furious when I arrived at his house that evening.

"How long's he been smoking cannabis?" His tone was accusing as he rose from his chair.

"Not that long, I don't think." I shrank beneath his glare. "What do I know? I don't bloody give him it!"

"I'm not having it!" His finger wagged in the air, not particularly at me but at the universe in general! "I want to know where he's getting it from! He's thirteen years old, for God's sake!"

* * *

"The little swine has pinched eleven quid off me!" Martin alleged that evening, slapping his wallet down like a prized fish on the kitchen worktop.

"Are you sure?" My stress levels began to rise as I stirred my drink.

"Sarah, it was all I had in it." He thumped his hand onto the soft leather of his wallet as though the action reiterated his point.

"Maybe you've made a mistake." I flung my teaspoon into the sink. Despite all we were going through, I never wanted to admit the worst about Tom until I had to.

"It was only last night when I checked it to make sure I didn't have to go to the bank. I've just opened it to pay for something in the shop, to find it empty." Snatching it up again, he thrust it before my face. "It was bloody embarrassing! So unless *you've* taken it, it must be Tom."

"I don't think he'd steal off you." Walking away from him, I was irritated that his immediate assumption was Tom was guilty of the theft.

"Oh come on!" He could not conceal his exasperation at the fact I was defending him. "It wouldn't be the first time, would it?"

Unfortunately, the allegation proved to be correct. Martin coerced the truth out of him later that evening by pretending the wallet had been fingerprinted! I ignored the smug look he gave me after Tom had flounced out of the room.

As a consequence, we attempted to ground him but he just roared with laughter into our faces before storming from the house anyway.

The First Arrest

August 2007 (13 years, 8 months)

"Tom's been arrested," Martin informed me flatly.

"What?" I gasped down the telephone, hoping I was dreaming the conversation.

"He's thieved a crate of beer from a shop. The stupid idiot thought he could pick it up and just stroll off with it." He laughed then, which irked me. "His mates did a runner and abandoned him to face the music."

After making my excuses at college, I began my reluctant journey to the police station.

"You've got my son in custody," I shakily announced to the desk sergeant. "Thomas Clifford."

"Ah yes." He scanned the 'admissions' board. "I must say, they're getting younger, these delinquents!"

I was led to the airless "custody suite." It was grim. Green, everywhere. Doors, walls, even the huge desk area which housed several police personnel. They regarded me as though I had committed a crime myself. Shuffling uncomfortably from one foot to the other, I was unsure where to look. I tried to close off my sense of smell to the overriding stench of odorous feet. Glancing down, I could see it was emitting from the numerous pairs of trainers that obediently waited outside the doors of the cells.

An officer unlocked one of the cell doors. Out crept my bleary-eyed son, appearing as though he might have been crying. As he avoided eye contact with me, I was amazed to notice what could have been shame crossing his face. I overcame the compulsion to hug him and glared at him instead.

"You stupid boy, what were you thinking of?" I demanded as I looked up into his face, suddenly realising that he now towered above me.

"I know." His gaze remained at his feet. "I won't do it again."

"I hope it's taught you a lesson, being banged up in there." I gestured in the direction of the cell from which he had just emerged.

"Not nice places, the cells, are they Tom?" grunted the officer, bashing information into a computer behind the green desk.

Tom shook his head. "I won't do it again. I'm sorry Mum."

"We're going to let you go with a caution this time," announced the officer. "But we never, ever want to see you in here again. Do you understand?"

"You won't!" I led him towards the door by the arm. "I'll make damn sure of that."

"What in God's name were you doing?" I reversed out of the car park.

"I fancied a drink." His smirk said it all.

"You're thirteen years old! You shouldn't be anywhere *near* alcohol, let alone pinching it!"

"Yeah right." Clearly his meekness in the police station had all been an act.

"Well, you're grounded all week and don't ask me for a single penny either. Your pocket money is well and truly stopped until further notice!"

He did stay in the following evening, but the one after, he ignored my protestations and strode out whilst I had my hands in the washing up bowl. I resisted the urge to chase after him. If I had captured him, I would not have been accountable for my actions!

It was approaching midnight when he fell in through the door. Anxiously, I had waited for him.

"You're drunk!" I shrieked, inhaling the stale stench that emitted from him.

"So what!" Slurring his words, he knocked into the banister at the foot of the stairs.

"Where did you get it from?" Grabbing his jacket, I tried to get him to turn and face me.

"Me mates." Placing his foot on the first step of the stairs was presenting a challenge for him.

"Look at the bloody state of you! You can barely walk! We'll discuss this in the morning!"

Laughing raucously, he lurched upwards. Soon after, I peeked into his room, relieved to find him sleeping. Gently placing a bucket beside him, I watched him sleep for a moment, making sure he was breathing OK. Just like I had when he was tiny. Still he looked the picture of innocence. My boy. The cause of constant angst and torment. When was it going to end?

His 'Friends'

September 2007 (13 years, 9 months)

Tom had acquainted himself with a rather undesirable bunch of friends. They would all hang about near our home, turning the air blue with their language. It was easy to see how Tom's behaviour had found itself in freefall again.

There seemed to be a lot of in-fighting between them. Once Tom surged through the front door as though he had the devil after him. Locking it, he then bolted upstairs. Within moments, a thumping at the door pursued him.

"Where is he?" demanded a pock-marked teenager, as I threw the door open.

"Upstairs." Standing with my hands resting on my hips, I counted five of them.

"I want him down here!" A youth at the back barged to the front and squared up to me, threatening my bubble of personal space.

"I think you'd better calm down first." I stepped back away from him.

"Get him down here now!" Another youth demanded from the back.

"Don't talk to me like that!" I started to feel anxious.

"And you're going to stop us are you?" mocked another, grinning around at his friends.

"Get away from my door!" I grappled for the handle. "Now!" As one tried to jam it open using his foot, I had to force its closure. I quickly locked it before racing upstairs. A loud hammering echoed in my ears.

"Whore!" One of them hollered from beyond the door.

I felt surprisingly scared. *Thank God Alex was asleep! And where was Martin when I needed him?*

"What's going on?" I demanded of Tom, who was observing his 'friends' from behind his curtain. They were hurling stones and clumps of mud at our house.

"One of em smacked me." Turning away from the window, he looked at me. "For no reason. They were filming it on a phone."

Taking hold of his chin, I studied his face. "Well you don't look as though you've been smacked."

"I got away, didn't I?" He jerked his chin away.

One of them then hollered the hideous expletive I had previously been called. I winced with its force.

"Have you heard what they're calling me?"

"It's not my fault." He returned to his curtained surveillance.

"They're your bloody friends."

I went to check on Alex, who miraculously still slept. Then I rang Martin. Whilst awaiting his answer, the front door clicked shut. Shooting to the window, I was not swift enough to see which way Tom had headed.

"Martin I need you to get home." Lifting my hand to my forehead was not going to miraculously ease my emerging headache. "Alex's in bed and I don't know what's going on around here. I need to find Tom; those lads might beat him up or something."

"He's a big boy now. He's probably brought it on himself anyway. You know what he's like."

For ten minutes, I fretted as I paced the lounge, before deciding that I must do something. Locking Alex in, I left the house to search for Tom. I only walked ten yards before I spotted him, striding towards me, thankfully unscathed.

"They'll regret it if they come at me again." Tom looked defiant as he patted his sock.

"What're you on about?" I grabbed hold of his shoulder as he sprang back up.

"They'll really get it." He widened his eyes, knowingly.

Then it dawned on me. "What have you got down your sock?"

"Nothing." He jutted his lip out defiantly.

"Show me. Now."

"I wasn't going to do owt with it." Bending down, he produced my vegetable knife which glinted antagonisingly in the early evening sunshine. A feeling of dread crawled over me.

"What if you'd fallen?"

"Well I wouldn't have done, would I?" He raised his eyes to the heavens.

"Tom, you're so stupid sometimes! What would've happened if the police caught you with it?" Shedding my cardigan, I then wrapped it around the knife. "You know all about knives! I don't understand you. What on earth were you going to do with it?"

"Just scare em." His tone lilted upwards as though I should have known that all along.

"And what if they'd grabbed it and turned it on you! I can't believe it, I just can't." I was ranting now but I didn't care.

The next evening his 'friends' returned. Rather than knock on the door, they rhythmically thumped upon it.

It was time for a new approach. Flinging the door open, I counted four of them this time.

"Where is he?" One of them demanded.

"Look lads," I tried, thinking I might have more success if I addressed them levelly. "What's the problem? You were all mates a couple of days ago, there's no need for all this trouble."

"He's a liar." An angry finger jabbed towards me.

"Look, I'm sure it can all be sorted out."

"We don't wanna talk to you. We wanna talk to him." He tried to peer beyond me.

"Tom's not here."

"Don't believe you." The youth attempted to swing the door open wider to get a better look.

"He's at his dad's."

"Well I wanna check his room to make sure." He took a step towards me.

I felt flabbergasted as I put my hand up to prevent him. "You're not getting one foot into my house. I've tried to be reasonable with you all but you just seem to want trouble." I began closing the door. "I don't know what Tom has done to upset you but you've no right to come banging on *my* door, giving *me* grief. I've a five-year-old in here. You're not being fair."

I shut the door on their mocking laughter, praying they would go away. Martin was at home this time, having a bath so I did not feel so vulnerable.

To assure myself of their complete departure, I stole a glance through the window and was horrified to find them spitting at my car and bombarding it with mud. Without thinking, I darted out towards them.

"Get away from my car or I'm calling the police," I screeched as they scattered like birds away from the car.

One of them screamed their favourite word at me; "whore!" As I scurried towards them, they all started running. Why they ran, I'm no sure, but I was relieved they did. If they had remained steadfast, I have no clue how I might have dealt with it.

They finished up behind a fence. I was not afraid of them, just furious.

"Do you not have any different words in your vocabulary?" I jeered as one of them repeated the previous expletive yet again! "That one's becoming tedious!"

"Sarah!" Martin roared as he strode towards me, with a face like thunder. At that moment the gang dispersed in all directions.

"Whatever were you thinking?" He caught up to where I stood. "They have weapons and all sorts these days! Don't *ever* put yourself in that position again!"

"My car," I panted. We both looked towards it where it languished, coated in disgusting spit and clumps of mud.

"Look, we'll sort it out tomorrow," he promised as he steered me back towards the 'safety' of our home.

Bittersweet

Elizabeth and Peter had news when I collected Tom that weekend.

"Tom's going to have a brother or sister!" Elizabeth patted her belly as she smirked at me.

"Congratulations!" I threw my arms around her. They had been together for years and I was aware of how badly she had wanted a baby of their own. But, try as I might, later that evening, I could not quell the nagging, intrusive and some might say; selfish thoughts.

What if they stop having Tom as often?

What if he wants to live with them full-time when they become a 'proper' family?

What if he bullies his new sibling as much as he's bullied Alex?

What if he dotes on his new sibling? How will Alex feel then?

Will Elizabeth still be as supportive when she has got a baby of her own?

Niggling, conflicting questions. A deep-seated suspicion that the worst might be yet to come with Tom. A knowledge that of course their priorities would lie with their unborn baby. A resentment that Peter was possibly going to sideline his eldest child in favour of his new one. A worry that I would soon be grappling for survival on my own.

Fortnightly

Before long, due to the decline in Tom's behaviour, Peter and Elizabeth reduced his weekly visits to fortnightly ones. It was hardly fair on Elizabeth to be expected to cope with such angst as she progressed through her pregnancy. One evening she rang me.

"Sarah, Tom's been using my bank card to credit his phone."

"Are you sure?" Raking my fingers through my hair, I screamed inwardly.

"Positive. I've been in touch with my bank. It's credited his number five times in the last few weeks."

Are you sure it wasn't Peter doing it for him?" *There I was, refusing again to believe the worst of him.*

"I've already checked that. That was the first thing I did. No. Tom's taken it upon himself to thieve money from me." Her voice rose up an octave. "At a time when I have everything to buy for the baby.

"I'm sorry. I really am. What do you want me to do with him?"

"Well. I've passed on his details to the bank. Whether they involve the police or not: I don't know. But we should make him believe that they will." I could hear the anger quivering in her voice. "He can pay it back to me as well."

We never discussed how this 'payback' might manifest itself. Perhaps I was expected to deduct it from his pocket money, subsequently taking the flack from him. Or maybe they were planning to reduce my maintenance payments. Privately, I thought he should do jobs in recompense. A fine idea in theory. This particularly episode spelt the beginning of the end for the respite that had been a necessity for me over the years.

Monthly

December 2007 (13 years, 11 months)

"He's asked what would happen to the baby if he was to boot me in the stomach!" Elizabeth shrieked at me down the phone. "He wanted to know if the baby would die!"
"Oh my God! Where's Peter?"
"Working. I can't cope anymore! *I just can't cope!"* She was hysterical.
"I'll come and get him." Wrenching mine and Alex's coats from their hooks, I then snatched up my car keys. "I'll be there in ten minutes."
"If I lose this baby because of him......"
I felt desolate as I made the brief drive. *How could he say such a thing?* I glanced at Alex, journeying in the passenger seat beside me, nearly six years old, calm and amenable. Every time I looked at him, I thanked my lucky stars. As for Tom, I'd be fortunate if they ever had him to stay again!
"Do you think I'm going to let you do to my baby what you've inflicted on HIM?" Elizabeth screamed at Tom, gesturing towards Alex upon our arrival.
"Calm down Elizabeth. Please!" I steered her towards her sofa. "You shouldn't be getting into this state! I'll take him home and sort him out. You get your feet up." I moved the footstool towards her. "This'll never happen again."
"Damm right it won't."
Later that day I received a text message to say they were reducing his visits to monthly ones. Slumping wearily onto the sofa, I silently contemplated the reality of *never* having a break from his antics. I was truly out of my depth.

"Mummy, I can smell smoke!" Alex screwed up his nose later that evening. So could I. Smoking was banned in our house. Mainly because of Alex's asthma but I also found the stink nauseating.

The swine was puffing away inside his bedroom. Taking the stairs, two at a time, I burst through his door.
"YOU DO NOT SMOKE IN MY HOUSE!"
"It's my room. I'll do what I like," Exhaling deeply, he then tapped his ash onto the carpet.
You won't!"
As I lunged towards the offending cigarette, he blew the smoke into my face, raging something unrepeatable. The hairs seared on my neck as I decided to back away. There would be nothing to gain from losing it. Besides I was in utter shock at the level of venom spewing from his every pore.

All I had ever done was love and take care of him. *How could he despise me so much?*

The next time I went upstairs, I paused as I heard money jangling. He was in Alex's bedroom, emptying his money box. I caught him in time though, saving the modest amount of money he had accumulated for his next batch of toy cars.

"Morning," smiled my neighbour as we both left our homes the next morning.
I fished around in my handbag for keys as we wandered together to our cars. "Morning, how are you?"
"OK thanks, has your week got off to a good start?"
"Not really." I was so upset that something I would not normally divulge to my neighbour just came tumbling out. "I've just caught my eldest trying to steal from my purse."
"Oh no!" She screwed her face up in sympathy.
"He seems to be going through another horrendous phase. I'm gonna have to start keeping everything out of his way."
"It sounds like you ought to fix locks on your doors."
"That might not be a bad idea."
Before long, that is how we began to live. Valuables locked away and my handbag always perched upon my shoulder. It became our normality. My friends were amused when I even kept

my bag about my person when I visited *their* homes. This 'bag attachment' was becoming ingrained!

When Alex came to open his cards on his sixth birthday, he discovered the task had already been performed. Tom had stolen all the money from them. After ringing around to find out who had put what in the cards, we discovered that his theft totalled £40. The people concerned promised they would give Tom's birthday money which was also approaching to Alex instead.

"How could you do that?" I waved the torn envelopes in his face.

"What does *he* need money for anyway?" Tom snatched them from me. "He's only six!"

"How dare you open other people's cards?" Wrenching a cup from the cupboard, I slammed it on the kitchen worktop. "You disgust me!"

"Shut up, you stupid fucking div!"

You may or may not agree with my actions but I swung a slap at him. However he was quicker than me and managed to dodge it.

Within days, he slipped into our bedroom and helped himself to our TV satellite box.

"What did you get for it?" I made no attempt to omit the sarcasm from my voice.

He ignored me.

"Where did you sell it?"

He shrugged his shoulders. In the same heist, we also discovered Martin's wedding ring had vanished. But Tom was admitting to nothing. We vowed that we could no longer afford lapses of forgetting to secure the bedroom door. Everything of value *had* to go in there. To have a thief living within our midst was heartbreaking.

The Behaviour Contract

January 2008 (14 years, 1 month)

As the school term recommenced, a meeting with Tom's head of year, Mr Wharton, was thrust upon me.

"I felt it was important to get something in place before Tom returns to lessons." he explained.

"Like what?" My voice echoed around the empty science lab with the remnants of potassium permanganate, sulphur and extinguished bunsen burners.

"Well, we know that it makes things tricky for you when we exclude him." He rummaged around in a file, "so we're going to try some other methods."

I was all ears. It was a huge relief that school acknowledged my predicament.

"Firstly, we're going to put him on a behaviour contract," he announced, finally stumbling across the correct sheet of paper. "It will involve me closely monitoring him."

"How will you do that?" I smiled, leaning precariously forward on the high stool to study it. "I've been trying that all his life!"

"Firstly, he'll have to come to me at the start of every morning *and* afternoon." He took out another sheet, which showed a shoddy attendance record. "Obviously I need to verify that he's actually in school."

I nodded, trying not to gasp at the 56% figure which blared out from it. "You do know I'm doing everything I can to get him here."

"Of course. I've seen you dropping him off on many a morning!"

"I bring him right up to the door," I added. "But I can't control what happens after that."

"I know. I agree with you."

"So why do I keep getting letters from Education Welfare, threatening me with further action?"

"I wouldn't worry about that. They're standard letters. If anything comes of them, we'll sort it. Anyway, back to this contract." He pointed at his sheet. "We're going to give him clear rules about the conduct expected in each lesson. His teachers will fill this form in at the end of every lesson to show whether he has achieved each target." He slid it over the workbench for me to inspect.

Arrive on time for lesson.
Stay in lesson.
Complete work set.
Display respectful and appropriate behaviour.

"But that's what he can't understand!" I stated as I gestured to the bottom 'target.' *Respectful and appropriate behaviour.* It needs to be more specific."

"We're going to do work with him around that. Miss Hussain, head of his *next* year group, also leads pastoral care." He gestured with his hands as he spoke. "She'll work on a one-to-one basis for at least two hours each week with him, to look at aspects of his behaviour and how it affects others."

"And when he breaks the contract?"

"He'll be dealt with using an *internal exclusion*. This is an effective deterrent for many pupils. Come with me, I'll show you the room." Rising from his stool, he replaced the sheets in the folder and grabbed his bag.

Obediently, I followed him to a room containing several wooden, graffiti-covered booths, not dissimilar to a polling station. It was airless and musty with an overwhelming smell of stale chewing gum.

"They hate it in here." Smiling, he swept his gaze over the room. "But if he can't work in class, he'll be working in here more often, supervised of course."

"And if that doesn't work?"

"We'll cross that bridge when we come to it."

My first contact with Miss Hussain did not begin on a good note. One morning, she was waiting for me when I dropped him off at school. A tiny Asian lady, she had a brisk manner and a stern voice.

"A mobile phone's been stolen from another pupil." She led me into her office.

"And it's Tom?" I glanced back at Tom before following her in, hoping that we would remain in the reception area as Miss Hussain had instructed. If left unattended, he had a habit of running off.

"There's no actual evidence, but his name *is* being banded about. Can you keep a look out for it?" Her voice was highly pitched and she was dressed in traditional Asian clothing sporting garish colours. "Maybe you could check his room at home?"

"Of course I will. I certainly wouldn't put it past him. He's light fingered enough at home. I can't even leave my handbag around anymore."

"I've been told all about it," her voice seemed to soften. "It sounds like you're having a tough time with him!"

"I always have had."

"I've been reading a bit of the background from his file. But I have faith that we can sort him out." I was surprised then at the change in her face as it unexpectedly broke into a smile. "He's not a bad lad deep down."

Even though I remained silent, my expression must have spoke volumes.

"I haven't failed *yet* with a pupil that's been allocated to me," she added, with an air that was aloof. We just need to bring out the best in him; give him opportunities to engage in things he excels at."

"Whatever you think." *Good luck,* I yearned to add.

"There's no such thing as 'bad' children." Looking curiously into my face, she seemed to be silently appraising me. "And Tom's certainly not one."

"How well do you know him?" *Surely she must have been kept up to speed with his antics at school.*

"Well.....we've had one or two encounters." She smiled; clearly the memory of these 'encounters' had provided her with a source of amusement. "But he's always polite."

"Well, I wish the same could be said of him at home." That morning's expletives were still echoing around in my head. "He speaks to me like I'm something he's stepped in."

Keep your Handbag on your Shoulder!

One morning, I left my bag in the kitchen. Tom was in there, like a rocket-fuelled turbo. I think I felt, rather than heard the abrupt movement. Anyway, I caught him in time.

"Well I needed some money." As I sidled into the kitchen, he snatched his hand away from my bag.

"Why didn't you just ask for some?" Glaring at him, I waited for his answer with my hands upon my hips.

He scowled. "Cos you're a tight cow!"

"You can't speak to me like that!"

"I just did." His next word was more offensive as he ascended the stairs.

My anger dissipated beneath a wave of sadness. *How can he speak to me like he does? I'm his bloody mum!*

Within moments, my thoughts were disturbed by the force of Alex's screeches.

I raced upstairs to find him clutching his face.

"What have you done?" Screaming at Tom, I hurtled towards Alex. Pushing past me, he tore down the stairs. The powerful scent of Martin's aftershave lingered in the air.

"I hate the lot of you!" Tom banged the door with such might that the house shuddered.

"He squirted me!" Alex refused to remove his hands from his eyes. He was obviously in agony.

Steering him towards the bathroom to get a towel, I noticed the discarded bottle of aftershave in Tom's bedroom doorway. *He'd squirted Alex's eyes with it.*

Quickly I filled the sink and bathed Alex's eyes with a flannel. He squirmed in pain as I dabbed at them. "You poor little thing. There, let's keep doing this. They'll soon stop stinging."

Missing

February 2008 (14 years, 2 months)

Although only fourteen years old; it was not out of character for Tom to stay out until all hours of the night.

On the first few occasions, I reported him missing if it got beyond midnight. The police would arrive; usually surveying me with an air of disgust before studying his photograph. They would scribble down a description and leave, informing me that an eye would be kept out for him as they went about their duties. He would always turn up though.

Once he returned whilst the police were taking his details, which pleased me. Sitting back, I smugly listened as they outlined the more important jobs they should be doing, rather than wasting their time and energy on a boy who didn't have the respect for his mother to return home when he was supposed to.

Eventually I stopped reporting him missing when he was late. Deep down I knew he was alright. I knew I would sense if he wasn't.

One Saturday morning I awoke with a start.

"Have you let Tom in during the night?" I nudged at Martin's sleeping form.

A negative response was grunted. I leapt out of bed and towards Tom's room, in case he had gained entry using alternative methods. He no longer had a key, having lost so many. Usually we concealed the key outside for him if he was likely to be home first.

His bed had not been slept in. Forcing myself not to panic, I reasoned in my mind that the selfish toad would be asleep at a friends. He would come back later, like always.

Only when dusk began to fall again, did I allow myself to panic. I rang his dad, two of his friend's mobile numbers that I found in his room and finally, the police.

"Why are you only *just* reporting him missing?" The policewoman surveyed me curiously, as though I was the most inadequate mother on the planet.

There was no sign of him that night either. By morning, I was worn out from pacing the house. I was driving myself demented by worrying what might have happened to him.

"All he has to do is ring me!" I wailed to Martin, staring through the window for the millionth time. "Just to let me know he's alright! I think something's happened." I stopped as this realisation crept over me. "He's never stayed out for this long before!"

It was difficult to act normally for Alex's sake. By lunchtime I decided it was time to go looking myself. Driving round every nook and cranny of the neighbourhood, I tried to pause alongside gangs of youths so I could inconspicuously scan their faces. From the back, they all looked like Tom, even the girls in their hooded 'uniforms.'

As dark fell again, a blanket-like depression wrapped itself around me. No way could I return home without him. Filling my car with more petrol, I then forced myself to wolf a packet of crisps before widening my search.

The groups of youths seemed more formidable in the dark. In desperation however, I began to stop and question them as to whether they knew Tom or had seen him over the weekend.

Most of them regarded me as though I was an alien species. My questioning produced a mixture of giggles and sarcastic responses. Nevertheless, one or two, mainly girls, seemed mildly sympathetic. But no one admitted to knowing of him.

Eventually, I struck lucky. "Yeah I saw him last night," slurred a girl, glancing at her friends as she spoke, as though she was seeking their approval. "He stopped at Meddy's gaff."

"Would you mind telling me where he, or is it a she, lives?" I plucked my phone from my bag, ready to type the information in.

She looked me up and down, suspiciously. "You say you're his mum, right?"

"Yes. All day I've been looking for him. I've even reported him missing. All I need to know is that he's OK."

Eventually she provided a street name, but claimed not to know the number. Within five minutes, I was there after punching it into my sat nav. After driving up and down several times, I spotted him with two people.

"Tom!" I wound down the window.

"Oh no, it's me mum." His companions sniggered. Tom tried to bolt behind a gate but swiftly realised there was no escaping me. "I'll be home later, right?"

"No it's not alright. Get in this car. NOW!"

"Get lost!" He reddened as his friends continued to laugh at him. "Do one!"

"Do you know? He hasn't been home since Friday. Probably not even washed himself or changed his underpants!"

His companions laughed raucously. Tom marched over and slung himself into the passenger seat.

"You make a show of me like that again and I'll fucking …………."

He gave no explanation and offered no remorse for what he had put me through other than he "couldn't be bothered" coming home. Apologetic noises were afforded to the police though, when they came to speak to him.

"Bloody filth," he jeered as soon as they left before speeding to the kitchen in pursuit of food.

I rang Elizabeth and Peter to inform of his return. They had been concerned but not to the extent I had.

"He's really putting himself at risk," stated Elizabeth.

"I know. I suspect he thinks he's older than he is." I closed the living room door so he could not hear our conversation. "The cannabis smoking, the truanting, everything……..it can't go on. I'm so worried about him……..I've no control……he just won't listen."

After further discussion we decided that Elizabeth would make a referral to social services, asking for help again. After all, by virtue of his own behaviour, he was making *himself* vulnerable.

How could I keep him safe if I had no idea where he was half the time?

Playing With Fire 3

"We're going to have to exclude him." Mr Wharton had rung me, yet again.

"Why. What's he done this time?" I was becoming convinced that Tom was acting up on purpose; obviously exclusion was wholly preferable to school.

"He's set fire to a bin," he sighed. "The entire school had to be evacuated."

"Oh, for God's sake! But what happened to him being punished with the internal exclusions?" I was conducting the conversation in the college library and had far too much work to be having to go retrieving and babysitting *him!*

"This is far too serious. He's going to have to remain at home for the rest of the week, I'm afraid."

"Great." I gathered my papers together.

"Can I ask," questioned the school receptionist the following week, "Why Tom isn't wearing uniform?" Her manner was just as condescending on the telephone as it was in person.

"He was wearing it this morning." I had to think for a moment but yes! We'd had a right row over it!

"Well he isn't now. And this is happening far too often. One of his teachers has asked me to inform you."

"He must have taken a change of clothes in his bag." I decided not to take issue with her superior tone of voice; I could not be bothered. "I'll check his bag in future"

"Well, if you could."

Mornings had become a constant battle.

"I'm not putting that on," he would protest with exacting regularity.

"Tom, every other pupil in your school has to wear uniform. Why should *you* be any different?

"I'm not wearing it. Alright?"

Sometimes he concealed a change of clothes *beneath* his uniform. Or he would try to sneak clothes out with him. Within days, I was accustomed with what and where to check. So he devised craftier methods of overcoming any problem that stood in his way, such as hiding his bag outside. He *was* wearing what *he* wanted for school. For this and a multitude of other reasons, I detested mornings.

Neither of us were 'morning people' and would clash like cage fighters. As he was growing, so was the severity of his attitude. The abuse I got from him was inexorable. When he was enraged enough, he would punch holes in walls or trash crockery.

Then came the straw that threatened to break the camel's back.

March 2008 (14 years, 3 months)

<u>What might you expect to get when Mother's Day falls on your birthday?</u>
(i) flowers
(ii) chocolates
(iii) perfume
(iv) breakfast in bed
(v) a lazy day
(vi) A police hunt for your son after he burgles your next door neighbour

As we drove up our street, anxiety mounted. Police officers were encircling our home. Parking quickly, I raced over.

"What's happened?" I gasped as I reached a police woman. "I live here!"

"Burglary. We're looking for the occupants of 164. Two lads. They've got into number 166 through the back door. They've taken quite a bit."

Adrenaline coursed through my body like a swollen river.

"YOU!!" screeched the girl from next door suddenly as she hurtled towards us. "Your son! I was barricaded inside my room by them!" Wailing hysterically, she continued to scream accusation at me. "What sort of parent brings up a monster like him?"

"That's enough." The police officer caught hold of her by the arms that were flailing ever more in my direction. "Let's get you inside. We'll catch him, don't you worry. It's not his mother's fault. I'll be with you in a moment," she nodded towards me before vanishing into next door with the young girl, shrieking like a banshee.

What on earth had been going through his head? Unlocking our door, I then leaned wearily against the door frame. Moments later, the policewoman's voice pierced my desolate thoughts.

"Your neighbour wants to apologise," she announced, steering me into my house. "She was upset as I'm sure you can understand. It's all been a dreadful shock for her, but she's aware that blaming you isn't the answer.

"*She* hasn't done anything to apologise for." I held the living room door ajar for her.

"The forensics will be along shortly to take prints." She followed me. "There are cars out searching for him and his mate."

It didn't feel real.

"Do you have a recent photo of him?" She scanned her eyes over our living room. I gestured towards the one that had been taken the previous year at school.

"Handsome young man; isn't he?" she commented as I wrenched it from the wall and despondently passed it to her. "Any idea why he'd want to commit a burglary? Doesn't look the sort."

"It's nothing to do with how he's been brought up." She thrust his grinning image back at me. "I've done everything I can with him. He's been a nightmare."

"I can vouch for that." The father of the girl next door had returned and came up behind the policewoman.

"Sarah, we're not blaming you." He brushed past the policewoman and into the our living room. "Not one bit. We just want our stuff back. And obviously for him to be punished."

"What did they take?" I was hugely indebted for his kind attitude. Perching myself onto the arm of a chair, I waited for his response.

"Two lap tops, a camera, a mobile phone, a purse and a games console." His voice was calm. There was no blame in his eyes as he peered at me. I could detect something else though; pity.

"I'm so sorry..."

"It's *him* who should be sorry. You didn't burgle us."

Just then his daughter emerged behind him. "I shouldn't have yelled at you like that. It's just the whole thing was so frightening." Her dad draped a protective arm around her shoulders. "I don't even know how many lads were in the house. I was there on my own - they could've done anything to me."

"He'll get what's coming. I'll see to it personally." Never in my life had I felt so guilty.

Several hours later, he returned. "Where've you been?" I hardly dared to look at him.

He slung himself into a chair. "Nowhere."

"Do you want some dinner?" I lifted myself up and started towards the kitchen.

"Yeah, I'm starving." I left him channel hopping, in blissful ignorance that I knew anything.

His plate spun around and around on the microwave turntable as I observed it. The smell of roast chicken caused me to feel even more churned up than I already did. After permitting him a few minutes to eat, I made the call. In hushed tones, I spoke to the police from the kitchen. They arrived within minutes, just as Tom was finishing his meal.

"I'm arresting you on suspicion of burglary and false imprisonment." I listened, with revulsion, on the sidelines as he was given his rights and led away. My eyes could not meet his.

*

"We're ready to interview now," asserted a male voice over the telephone. "Can you make your way to the station?"

"Why?" That was the last place I wanted to be.

"As an appropriate adult. To ensure fair treatment for your son." His tone suggested I should already be aware of this. "It's standard procedure."

"So Tom receives the reassuring presence of his mother? I don't think so." No way could I sit at his side after what he had done. They enlisted the Youth Offending Team instead. It was hours before I heard anything further.

Eventually they telephoned me again. "We're releasing him. Your neighbour didn't physically see him; she just believes she recognised his voice amongst the others. There's no evidence to actually place him at the crime scene."

"But there must be fingerprints......" I could hardly face my neighbour as it was. But if he was to get away with this......

"None."

"You're joking!" My voice rose up. "But he did it!"

"We know that. However there's no proof to charge him. Only if he confesses."

"Right!" I snatched up my car keys from the coffee table. "Keep him there! I'm on my way!"

"Just do the right thing," I urged Tom in the sweltering green interview room. The officers had left us alone. He looked dishevelled and unbelievably childish. Being incarcerated for several hours had taken its toll.

"I just want them to let me go Mum. This place is awful." His bottom lip wobbled. For a moment I thought he was going to cry.

"Why did you do it?"

"We didn't plan it." Genuine regret momentarily seemed to seep into his expression. "The door was open and we both kind of egged each other on."

"But you locked her in her room." I shuddered to imagine what must have been going through the poor girl's mind whilst this was going on.

"I'm not proud of myself you know." He stared down at his hands.

Tom was unaware of the predicament and had no idea that the police did not have adequate evidence with which to charge him. At his still tender age, he would not have understood the technicalities anyway.

"If you're honest, you'll be in less trouble." I studied his face for his reaction.

"But they'll lock me up."

"Not if you tell the truth." I rested my hand on his arm. "You'll be punished, yes, but they'll go easier on you if you own up to what you've done."

"And then will they let me go." His eyes glimmered hopefully.

"Yes and I'll stay with you this time whilst they interview you."

The police obtained a taped confession for which they thanked me. He and his friend were charged and released on bail, with a curfew to be in at home between seven at night and seven in the morning.

Some mums might have felt guilty but there was no way I would have wanted him to get away with his actions; I felt satisfied with what I had done. The looming punishment would act as a future warning as no sanction I ever meted out seemed to improve his behaviour: maybe the courts would be more successful?

The Third Arrest

"We're arresting you for criminal damage ...."

I closed my eyes as Tom was marched from our house by the police two days later.

There was no denying his actions that had been captured on CCTV. This time I agreed to act as his 'appropriate adult' at the station.

They also quizzed him regarding a recent break-in that had occurred in an adjacent street to where we lived, but had insufficient evidence with which to charge him.

After his interview, I was told to wait in the public area whilst the Crown Prosecution Service suggested the next course of action.

Beleaguered, I slumped onto the freezing metal seat that was screwed to the floor. Whilst surveying the bleak surroundings, I tried to avoid meeting anyone else's gaze. Thirty minutes were whiled away sending off text messages to various people.

Just as I started to wish I had brought something to read, my thoughts were broken into by the officer who had interviewed him.

"We need you to be present whilst we search him." His head popped around the door into the waiting room.

"Search him?" I jumped up, my backside numb from the lengthy wait. "But haven't you already done that?"

"I'm afraid we need to *strip search* him this time?" Looking sheepish, he guided me back to the custody area. "He's stowed smoking paraphernalia where the sun don't shine. We need to ensure he hasn't got anything else concealed up there."

For the first time in my life, I witnessed the interior of a cell. I didn't know where to look as they did the necessary. Although I was supposed to be present, I did my upmost to linger outside the cell door.

"Are you queer or summat, you?" Tom's words made me wince as I hopped from one foot to the other. He was certainly doing himself no favours!

"We'll give these to you for safekeeping," announced the officer, as he led me away from the cell, thrusting the lighter and cigarette he had retrieved towards me.

"Ugh! You must be joking!" I hid my hands behind my back. "Throw them in the bin!"

They decided to tie the criminal damage case in with the burglary, to be dealt with together at court. I would receive a call when I could return to collect him. It had been decided to keep him locked up a bit longer because of his attitude!

A letter waited for me on the doormat when I arrived home:

4th March 2008
Dear Tenant,

We refer to the unfortunate incident perpetrated by your son on 2 March, which has been just brought to our attention.

In the interests of all concerned, we would regrettably ask that you make suitable arrangements for your family to vacate the property at your earliest convenience.

We would ask that you contact this office to discuss a timescale in which this can take place.

Yours faithfully

Housing Officer

It was about five hours later that I got the call from the police station.

"The CPS has allocated a court date," announced a young male voice. "Tom will be on a seven o'clock curfew at your property until after then. You can come and collect him now." It was approaching eleven o'clock at night.

"I'm not collecting him." I'd drunk wine by then and was in no frame of mind to confront Tom after the letter I'd had.

"You're his appropriate adult," his voice grew stern. "You *must* collect him."

"I don't want him here."

"Well, I'm not being funny but we don't want him here either. He's taking up a cell!"

"I'm going to lose my home because of him!" Tears were dripping from my eyes. I tasted their salt as I opened my mouth to speak. "I've had enough."

"Look, love," his voice softened slightly. "Is there anyone else who could pick him up?"

I shook my head, forgetting I was on the phone.

"What about his father?"

"He's just had a new baby with his girlfriend. *He* won't be able to come."

"Look love......"

"Stop calling me love!" I must have sounded unhinged!

"He's your son, your responsibility; you must come and collect him. NOW!"

"You might as well ring social services. I've had enough. I can't cope with him anymore." I shook as I spoke. It was either with exhilaration or exhaustion. Or both.

"Are you saying you won't have him back?"

"That's exactly what I'm saying!" It was exhilaration. Suddenly, I felt empowered.

"You can't do that!"

"Watch me." I was finally making a stand!

"Well I've never come across anything like this before. I'll have to speak to my superiors."

At that moment, I realised that I *did not* want him back. I couldn't take anymore. Silently, I left the police officer to ponder the predicament as I gently replaced the receiver.

Weeping silently, I awaited the outcome of our conversation. Within ten minutes the phone sprang back into life. I ignored it. Then I ignored it again. All was calm for about twenty minutes. I pictured my son, sitting in the cell and tried to feel guilty about the confusion and rejection he would be feeling, but I couldn't.

They would have rung social services by now. A social worker would be on their way to pick him up; maybe they would put him in a care home, or perhaps with foster parents. Whichever, they would definitely have their work cut out with him.

My thoughts were disturbed by a hammering at the door before it was pushed ajar. Tom stood in the doorway; a mixture of defiance and tiredness.

"We made a call to social services." The police officer nudged Tom towards me. "We were told to return him home. *You* have a duty of care." He pointed at me. "If you try to pull that stunt again, we'll prosecute. Do you understand?"

I nodded dismally, unable to raise my gaze from my feet.

"Somebody from social services'll be out to see you," he continued, backing away. "But they won't be taking him into care. You can forget that!" He seemed to laugh slightly but it sounded more like a sniff. "He's all yours!"

Didn't I know it?

School Exclusion

The court date was a month away. In the meantime, he was excluded from school again; this time he had been *caught* stealing someone's phone.

"We're not sure if the girl's parents are going to involve the police," the school receptionist informed me in icy tones over the telephone. "Not now it's been found."

"Could you *ask* them to inform the police?" I leaned against a wall. "If he isn't punished, he'll just keep on stealing." I was on my break from a college lecture. Several people peered towards me when they heard me say 'police.' I flushed, self consciously.

"Right, I'll pass your wishes on." She paused, seemingly writing something down. "I've also been asked to tell you about yesterday. Tom's head of year meant to call you but hasn't had chance."

"Yesterday?" I moved myself from earshot of my audience.

"Yes, someone deliberately set the fire alarms off. The whole school had to be evacuated. During this time the deputy head had his phone stolen from the jacket he had been forced to abandon in his office."

"And Tom's taken that too?" Clearly they had him 'bang to rights' already!

"Well that's just it. We've no proof whatsoever. Several people saw him loitering around the deputy's office and that's where the fire alarm originated from but ……"

"I'll go through his bedroom before he comes back. But I have to say……I don't think he'd be daft enough to leave it anywhere where I'd find it."

Despite looking, the phone never surfaced.

Within days, we realised Martin's mobile from his expired contract had vanished from beneath our bed. At first we admonished each other for leaving the door unlocked; then we confronted Tom.

"It wasn't me," he stated, his blue eyes meeting mine and firmly fixing their gaze. "I'm not going to pinch from anyone anymore.

Especially from any of you Mum. I'm going to sort myself out, I promise." His face looked so earnest I almost believed him.

"Do you know I've rigged a video camera up in there," fibbed Martin, his expression silently daring me not to give the game away. "We've got you on it and we're going to let the police know."

"No, please, don't!" he begged. "I can't be banged up again!"

"Well you should've thought about that, shouldn't you?" Martin edged closer to him. "What've you done with it?"

"I've sold it."

"To who?"

"To a shop."

"What shop?"

"I can't remember." His eyes stayed fixed on his feet.

"Well we'll see if you can remember when the police ask you." Martin snatched up the telephone receiver.

Tom's response was a tirade of four letter words. After he had stomped from the house, I plucked the phone from Martin's hand. I knew if I postponed ringing the police, I would persuade myself out of it.

"I want to report a theft," I announced shakily upon connection.

As I gave further details, the operator seemed efficiently interested until she gleaned that the culprit was my fourteen-year-old son.

"Well it won't be put on as a priority," she informed me, curtly. "You'll receive a visit within two to three days."

It was actually four days, and the 'mighty' CPS decided not to pursue my complaint, anyway.

It seemed Tom was on a roll of 'getting away' with things.

Soon after, Martin took a phone call from an irate neighbour, also a mother of one of Tom's friends. It emerged that she had disturbed Tom and another lad breaking into her house.

Having been told by his friend that the entire household was going away, Tom had seized the 'opportunity' but had been misinformed of their date of return, meaning he had attempted to rob them in the belief they were still away.

They had scarpered as though their lives depended on it when they were caught in the garden. The woman asserted that she couldn't be bothered with the hassle of involving the police; however she wanted us to deal with him, and to also ensure he stayed well away from *her* son in the future.

Before he returned home, I confiscated his computer, knowing it would hurt him. It was the only thing that seemed to occupy his time whilst he was at home. It had the desired effect. Though the torrent of abuse I got wounded me just as much!

Social Services

I was taken aback by the arrival of not one, but *three* social workers at the appointed time. Perhaps this quantity of them was indicative of imminent support.

"We've received the referral from Tom's stepmum," announced the youngest looking of the three. And when I say young, I mean young! They perched on my sofa, in a line, their right legs primly crossed over their left. "I gather you're concerned about his vulnerability when he's out and about."

"Things have moved on since then," I informed her, balancing on the edge of an armchair. "He's now in trouble with the police."

"Yes, we've been made aware of that." Her voice was bird-like and she looked as though she's spent at least an hour applying her cosmetics. "It sounds as though he's putting you through it." The other two chuckled. I glared at them.

"I've been to hell and back with him actually." Unsure who I should be addressing, my gaze flickered between them. "And I feel as though I'm on my way back there again." They could no doubt detect the hostility within my voice so I consciously tried to load friendliness into it. "I need help."

"We've got his history on our files," asserted one of the 'chuckle sisters.' "And we've contacted school. I'm unsure as to what help *we* could offer though." *Typical. What you mean is you can't be bothered!*

"Anything! I just can't cope with him. He's bullying me *and* my younger son. I'll freely admit I've no control over him. I need this taking out of my hands. Surely this is where social services can step in?" My voice was cracking as I pleaded.

"Only with children at risk, *not* children with behaviour problems," affirmed the first social worker, glancing at her colleagues, perhaps for approval.

"But he *is* at risk. He's putting *himself* at risk! He's fourteen years old and he's using cannabis for God's sake! And not long ago, he did not even come home for three days!" My arms were flailing about with my words, as is they could add support to my plight. "I never know where he is!"

"Have you been ever been offered a parenting course?" *Bravo! The magical parenting course! The answer to all my problems!*

I laughed, drily. "I'd try anything if I thought it'd help. It's not me with the problem though."

"Could you give me a moment to speak with my colleagues please?"

Evidently, I was expected to leave the room. The uselessness of it all made me want to scream.

After vacating my living room, I strained to decipher the low hum of conversation for several minutes. Feeling utterly deflated, I accepted they weren't going to offer any assistance. *A bloody parenting course!* Then the main spokeswoman's head popped around the door.

"You can come back in now," she announced, all lipstick and heady perfume.

"Oh thanks." *Whose house was it?*

"We're going to give you a number." Reclining back between her colleagues, she rummaged in her designer shoulder bag. "You can ring it anytime you need to unburden yourself." The embossed card she shoved before me was emblazoned with a parenting helpline number. "There'll always be someone there to listen. Twenty Four hours a day." Easing herself back into the chair again, I got the impression she was revelling in a job well done.

"And that's it?" In disbelief, I stared at her.

"The help line's staffed by trained volunteers. Sometimes it helps to talk."

"I don't need that kind of help! I need respite or something."

"Look, all we can do is return to the office and consider whether there is anything further we can offer you." As if they were tuned into one another, they all rose simultaneously. "We'll be back in touch after we've liaised with our supervisor."

Useless! Useless! Useless!

The First Court Appearance

I persuaded Tom to wear trousers for court.

"It'll show respect," I assured him, ignoring his protestations against wearing a 'gay' pair of trousers.

Outside court, I noticed he was the only person in trousers and 'proper' shoes. Comparing him with the other youths; most of them seemed older and it felt surreal that Tom was being classified similarly. It was as though there was a dress code imposed: trainers, baggy tracksuit bottoms and hooded tops.

Disgrace shone from me whilst forced to stand before three magistrates and state my name beside him. His crimes of burglary, false imprisonment and criminal damage were dealt with together.

When we were eventually dismissed, he rejoiced. His *punishment* was reparation: a weekly appointment with the youth offending team.

I, on the other hand, was ordered to compensate our neighbour to the tune of £600. The criminal damage cost me £430. I was also 'awarded' court costs!

For the first time, I regretted my role in coercing him to own up. It was me being punished, not him! I had envisaged a stern amount of community service and some kind of victim awareness intervention for his crimes. The outcome had far exceeded my expectations.

Before we were allowed to leave court, we had to meet with a court liaison officer from the youth offending team. The side room we were shepherded into contained a poisonous looking, middle-aged woman. Her hair was lacquered to perfection but she had red lipstick all over her teeth. Had the circumstances been different, I would have alerted her to this make-up malfunction.

"Sit!" she growled.

As though I had been convicted myself, I dropped into the seat at her command. Cameras were positioned in every orifice of the room, yet people had been daring enough to daub the place in graffiti or carve their names into the table at which we now sat.

"So, let's have a look at you then." She peered at Tom across the table as though he were an insect. "Think you're a big man do you? Burgling; criminal damage; truanting from school; making your poor mother's life HELL!" I jumped as she screeched the final word.

Tom, for once, remained silent. "Do you know where you're going to end up?" Recoiling, I observed congealed spit escaping from the corner of her mouth. "I'll tell you shall I? A young offenders' institution. Where all no-hopers like you finish up."

"I'm not a no-hoper." Glowering, he avoided her gaze.

Go on, lose your temper Tom! She'll make mincemeat of you!

"Oh yes you are." Prodding at the table with her immaculately manicured fingernail, she continued. "I can see it in your eyes. You're like all the others. Think you can do what the hell you want. Well I've got news for you. You can't."

"I know I can't." Slouching back in his chair, he folded his arms. *Yeah, course you do!*

"Sit up straight when I'm talking to you!" She sucked up the drool that persisted in escaping from her crimson lips. "Do you know how fortunate you are to be sat here in front of me?"

Tom shook his head.

"Very fortunate." Slapping her palm against the table in front of him caused him to jump. "Very fortunate indeed. You should've left that courtroom by the other door and now be locked in the back of one of those prison vans. And next time, you will be." Smirking, she gave him a knowing stare.

"There won't be a next time." Tom's voice was softer than I'd ever witnessed and he sat bolt upright, seemingly not daring to twitch a muscle.

"There will be if you miss one of these appointments." She thrust two cards at him, which he proceeded to pass to me. "No, they're your cards!" She manoeuvred his arm out of my direction. "Your appointments." She poked an angry finger towards him. "Your responsibility. That one's a weekly appointment with your youth offending worker; the other is for your reparation."

"What's that?"

"You'll be doing unpaid work to show how sorry you are. Twenty hours." *Whoopee,* I scorned internally, *is that it?*

Meekly, he slid the cards into his pocket.

"Bye love," he muttered as we left. Knowing she would not be happy with that, I cringed.

"Don't *ever* call me love! Do you hear me?"

"Stupid bloody cow!" We closed the door behind us.

"Always the big man, aren't you Tom?" I half hoped she had heard him. "You wouldn't dare call her that to her face."

The Anti-Social Behaviour Contract

"This is the first step towards you receiving an anti-social behaviour order," stated the police officer. We had been summoned to the police station, where I had once again, to act in an 'appropriate adult' capacity for the implementation of his anti-social behaviour contract. The officer had a sheet of paper in front of him, which I strained to read, upside-down.

"You mean an 'asbo'?" Tom sounded happy at the prospect.

"You're incredibly young to have two convictions!" he growled. "Anyway, if you breach the terms of this order, you're risking your parent's tenancy and increasing the likelihood of fines they'll be responsible for."

"When does he get punished?"

"We expect *you* to take care of that." His glare was piercing, leaving me in no doubt as to his view of me.

"I've tried everything with him." I didn't want the police officer harbouring this opinion. I was fed up with everyone blaming me! "If I ground him, he climbs out of windows. If I stop his money, he steals. If I forbid him from doing something, he does it anyway."

"Not our problem." Leaning back, he wearily clasped his hands behind his balding head, revealing two stale sweat patches under his arms.

"It's not as if I'm a parent who doesn't 'give a monkeys.' I'm here aren't I? I want to sort him out. But I can't." It was fruitless trying to convince this man of anything. "I've tried asking for help but no one will give me any."

"Shut the fuck up Mum!" Tom jarred me with his elbow.

"Look, you can hear how he talks to me. What am I supposed to do?"

"We're going round in circles here, love." He checked his watch. "Let's just concentrate on the contract, shall we. I'll read it out."

ACCEPTABLE BEHAVIOUR CONTRACT

THIS CONTRACT is made on the 9th April 2008
BETWEEN YORKSHIRE POLICE
AND THOMAS CLIFFORD
THOMAS AGREES the following in respect of future conduct –

1. I will not write graffiti or damage any property in and around the Kirkwood area.

2. I will not take any property that does not belong to me.

3. I will not climb on any rooftops, lift shafts or any other prohibited areas.

4. I will not abuse residents or passersby. This includes swearing.

5. I will attend school.

FURTHER THOMAS enters into a commitment with YORKSHIRE POLICE not to act in a manner that causes or is likely to cause harassment, alarm or distress to one or more persons not in the same household.

Breach

If THOMAS does anything which he has agreed not to do under this contract which YORKSHIRE POLICE considers to amount to anti-social behaviour, an application may be made to the magistrates' court for an ANTI-SOCIAL BEHAVIOUR ORDER to prohibit THOMAS from acting in a manner likely to cause harassment, alarm or distress to one or more persons not of the same household.

DECLARATION

I confirm that I understand the meaning of this contract and that the consequences of breach of the contract have been explained to me.

SIGNED   Tom Clifford   Individual
DATE 9th April 2008
SIGNED   Sarah Pearson   Parent
DATE 9th April 2008
SIGNED   PC 4112 McIntyre   Police Officer
[Name of police officer]
DATE 9th April 2008

The Enemy Within

Cannabis usage was certainly driving Tom. He funded this addiction by stealing from our home. No longer, were any of us permitted to own money boxes and small change jars; he had pilfered them all. Frustrated by their non-replenishment, he would route around the house for money on a daily basis. His lack of success provoked frustration and outrage. We learned through bitter experience, never to leave valuables lying about.

I became surgically attached to my handbag as Tom would be straight in for my purse if it was left unattended. Once I fell asleep on the sofa and awoke to find £12 and my mobile phone missing.

"You should report it the police again," Martin declared upon arriving home.

"Look at the waste of time it was before!" I shook my head. "We'll have to deal with him ourselves. Stop his money for a while."

His pocket money never lasted long anyway. He became intolerable when it ran out. If his demands were not met, which they hardly deserved to be, holes would be punched in walls and doors. Or he would hurl whatever was to hand down the stairs.

One morning, Martin remembered his wallet which he had left in his coat pocket.

"Sarah, grab my wallet from my coat," he whispered from the bath. "I've just heard Tom get up. If he pinches from me, that's all I've got."

Slinking downstairs, I discovered Tom had beaten me to it.

"Give it here" I held out my hand.

"No." He fastened his fingers tightly around it. "Fuck off!"

Flying at him, I tried to prise the wallet from his grasp. *God, he was getting strong.*

"Get off, you piece of shit!" Then his voice hardened further. "Do you want a fucking slap?" His words stung me far more than a slap ever could.

Recoiling in horror, shock washed over me as I surveyed the fury on his pinched face. Just then, Martin's angry footsteps came bounding down the stairs. He seized Tom by the scruff of the neck.

"You ever pinch off us again, or abuse your mother in that way and I will have you!" Fragrant steam radiated from his shoulders into the air.

Tom stood steadfast, smirking defiantly, his upright middle finger conveying his unspoken thoughts. Martin flew back upstairs and slammed around for several minutes as he dressed. Then, evidently livid over the whole situation, he stormed out of the house without further comment.

"Where's he gone – I wanted a cig off him!" ranted Tom, his face contorted with rage as he watched Martin's car roar away.

"Just get a move on Tom. You're going to be late." Snatching up my car keys, I dropped Alex's coat into his lap. "I'll gift you a lift to the bus stop." The day had barely begun and I already felt as though I'd had enough.

"Oh yeah, and how am I supposed to have a smoke. Fucking idiot!" He banged out of the room.

"Hurry up Tom, we've got to go." I called up the stairs a few minutes later, desperately trying to quell the stress in my voice.

"Shut up you div," he sneered.

I blinked back the tears that were needling behind my eyes. It wasn't until I dropped Alex off at school that I finally unleashed them.

"I can't take it anymore!" Howling in the silence of the car, I punched the steering wheel. "I've had enough!"

Brought Home by the Police 1

May 2008 (14 years, 5 months)

"Is this your son?" The policeman unhooked his grip from Tom as he awaited my reply.

"You should be at school! Oh my God!" I stood, agape, as he collapsed through the doorway. "Look at the state of you!"

"We found him vomiting in the street. He's clearly under the influence of something but won't admit what." Rubbing his hands together as though he'd had hold of a decaying bird, he stepped back. "In view of his age, we had a duty to pick him up."

"Thanks," Tom began an attempt to ascend the stairs. I knew exactly what the 'substance' was and suspect the policeman did too. He stunk of it!

"Get yourself to bed Tom," he called after him. "Good luck," he nodded at me. "I trust you'll speak to him about this."

"Of course."

Another Bullying Incident, School Exclusion 5

June 2008 (14 years, 6 months)

"Sarah, it's Miss Hussain," announced the voice. "You'll have to collect Tim right away. We're going to have to say he can't return till after half term."

"But that's nearly three weeks!" I protested, quickly processing the implications of this exclusion in my mind. "What on earth's he done now?" I segregated myself from the friends I was having lunch with in the college canteen, not knowing them well enough to allow the gory details of my son's behaviour to be laid bare.

"He, along with his *girlfriend**, attacked another pupil."

"I didn't know he had a girlfriend." Ambling over to the window, I observed a huddle of students as they lounged about in the sunshine, seemingly without a care in the world.

"I shouldn't say this, but between you and me, she's not the nicest character, quite foul-mouthed, often in trouble."

"No wonder he's hooked up with her then. But who've they attacked?"

"I've been a teacher for nearly fifteen years. Never have I witnessed such a nasty assault on a fellow pupil. The two of them were booting her in the head. She was in agony. It took several members of staff to intervene and get them off her."

"She?" I screeched, forgetting where I was. Glancing around to check who was paying attention to me, I lowered my voice. "He's hurt a *girl*?"

"I'm afraid so. Her parents are in with the head teacher at the moment. I'm not sure what their course of action will be."

I was speechless for a few moments as I tried to digest the information. "Can you give them a message from me?"

"I'm not sure that's the best......"

"Just tell them how sorry I am." I slumped into a chair at an empty table. "Not just sorry. Gutted. Ashamed. Devastated." *The poor girl!* "Tell them to report him and his *girlfriend* to the police. I urge them." Several of my friends were peering across at me, no doubt speculating as to what on earth my conversation could be about. "He must be punished properly for this."

"I'll tell them. Thanks for being understanding."

"I just want what's right." I rested my head down onto the flat of my palm. "I can't believe it to be honest! How's the girl?"

"I'm not sure. She was hysterical and in a lot of pain. We're all in shock." Mrs Hussain sounded more subdued that usual. "Like I say, I've never witnessed such an awful incident within a school. We've no idea what provoked it."

After our conversation had ended, I rang Peter. "If I set eyes on him I won't be responsible for my actions," I wept, noticing that my friends were starting to move themselves in preparation for our next lecture. "Please will you collect him? I can't take anymore!"

"OK," he agreed flatly. "Though I don't know what you expect *me* to do with him. I'm only going to put him in his room and ignore him."

"Just make sure you remove his TV and games console first." I shuffled towards my original table
and gulped final swig of my now-cold tea.

"Too right."

Disappointingly, the girl's parents decided not to prosecute. They were satisfied with his exclusion. Later, I went to collect him from his dad's, not wanting to, but obviously having to.

"He's gone," asserted Peter, not breaking his gaze with the TV.

"What do you mean, gone?" I swung Tom's door open to be greeted by his curtains ballooning outwards against the gaping window.

"Great, so he's escaped. Now what're we supposed to do?"

"Not a lot we can do." Peter's face was heavy with suppressed anger. "Just wait for him to come back, I suppose."

*The 'girlfriend' did not feature with him for more than a couple of weeks, however in this time, he stole expensive perfume I had been given for my birthday for her.

All the Professionals (The Common Assessment Approach)

List of Agencies currently involved with young person

1. Youth Offending Team
2. Social Services
3. Positive Activities for Young People
4. Kirkwood Medical Centre
5. Child and Adolescent Mental Health Service
6. Fielding Park High School
7. Education Welfare

General Health

Tom is physically fit. He smokes cigarettes and cannabis. Mum has concerns about his drug
use and the impact this is having on his mental health. Mum says he suffered from ADHD when he was younger and still exhibits symptoms, i.e. lack of concentration, difficulty sleeping and destructive behaviour.

Tom has admitted he does smoke cannabis a few times a week (mainly at weekends) however
he feels that he does not need help from anyone regarding his drug use. He has had two sessions with 'Base 10 drugs information service,' and then decided to withdraw from these sessions.

Personal Development

Mum feels Tom responds better to male adults and demonstrates a lack of respect towards females. He has friends (usually older than himself, aged 16/17) and hangs around the streets with them. Mum feels that these friends also smoke cannabis.

She knows that she appears to be 'always getting on at him' which must have a negative impact on his confidence at times.

Dad and step mum, Elizabeth have recently had a baby and have restricted contact and visits due to his offending behaviour.

Mum feels that Tom has a real lack of self control and has real problems with his behaviour at home. He has also received exclusion on several occasions from school. His drug taking has led to offending behaviour and he is on a twelve month referral order with the youth offending team.

Enjoying and Achieving

Tom continues to truant from school and is receiving one-to-one support from the parental support officer and head of year. He will go off site and not return from lunch. He is brought into school each morning by step-dad, Martin. Tom is on a behaviour contract at school; however he continues to display challenging behaviour. Mum states his behaviour can be physical at home and he will 'smash things up' and 'punch the doors and walls.' Whilst he will apologise for his behaviour, Mum feels that he shows no emotion behind the apology. Mum is concerned that he does not show remorse for his actions, e.g. towards the victim after the recent break in of their next door neighbour. Tom says he disagrees with this and he does feel guilty about their impending eviction.

Parenting Examples

Mum is caring and consistent, however she feels 'out of her depth.' She sets boundaries and gives encouragement to Tom but feels powerless to make a difference.

Tom has been known to run out of the house and has gone missing on occasions. Mum feels like she has provided a stable home life for him; however his recent offending may result in the family being evicted from their current home. Mum feels that Tom has a better relationship with step-dad Martin, than with her.

Family and Environment

Tom no longer stays overnight with Dad and Elizabeth. Efforts on their part to maintain contact with him through meeting him in the town centre have been rejected by him.

Mum has to lock everything away in the house otherwise Tom will take it. Mum feels he sells these items to fund his drug addiction. He has also been known to sell his own clothes and his brother's play station games.

Mum feels Tom is heavily into drugs and feels this is a 'daily addiction.' She says he has no desire to stop these drugs and feels that this is linked to his criminal behaviour.

Work Together to name WHAT changes people want to see

- Increased attendance at school
- Stop criminal/antisocial behaviour
- Face up to drug use/problem
- To see a positive change in Tom's mood
- Tom to follow rules at home and come in on time at night

Tom's comments when consulted were 'He would like a motorbike.'

Record ideas on HOW to make this happen

- YOTS – work to be undertaken on drugs, anger management, victim awareness, community service
- PAYP – to invite Tom to positive activities
- CAMHS – Mum awaiting first appointment
- Social Services – feel there is no role for them at this time

Views
- Tom is OK with the Common Assessment Framework Approach but may not engage with professionals
- Mum is relieved she will receive additional support
- Tom is a young man with many problems and multi-agency input is the way forward.

The GP (again)

"It's about Tom again," I wearily informed the doctor as I plonked myself on the chair in front of her.

Sympathetically, she smiled at me. "No improvement then, I take it?" She had never judged me and had always empathised and tried to help. But short of referring us on elsewhere, I knew there was little she could do.

Shaking my head, I sighed heftily. "He's moving onto bigger and better things now. You know, stealing, truanting, criminal damage, cannabis, alcohol, that sort of thing."

Her expression drooped. "I hoped he'd grow out of it all."

"No chance." I clasped my hands together in my lap. "I'm not really convinced about this Conduct Disorder thing, you know. I think it's something else. If we could just get a diagnosis then maybe he could get treatment and maybe......."

"It's not as simple as that, Sarah," she rested her hand on my arm to stop me. "It never has been."

"I know, but I can't give up on him. I've got to keep trying."

"I think you've done an amazing job coping with it, all these years."

I brightened a little. "Thanks." It meant a lot, being acknowledged. "Can you refer us anywhere?"

"The 0-19 Team?" She whipped a pen from her desk.

I groaned. "Isn't there anywhere else?"

Her face conveyed her powerlessness. "With these sorts of problems, they always have to be the first port of call. Hopefully, they'll be able to refer you on though."

"Here we go again."

This time the 'assessment' was to occur over three sessions, due to his now advanced age.

I, with Elizabeth's backing, placed every problem we were experiencing at the man's well-heeled, polished feet, expecting him to have some solutions. By now, going over and over the same information repeatedly was tedious.

"I just want a diagnosis and medication for him," I informed the man, scanning his face for a flicker of sympathy or understanding. "There *is* something wrong with him. There always has been."

"We'll have to get him reassessed by a child psychiatrist," stated the man, suddenly seeming to jerk into life. "I gather he's seen one before."

I sat up straight. It *had* helped last time. He must have noticed my downtrodden body giving way to sudden optimism.

"I'm not promising they'll find anything mind." He wagged his finger at me. "Mental health problems in adolescents are notoriously difficult to establish."

"I know. But I want them to try."

"He'd also have to be willing to co-operate." The man's pen lingered over the referral form he was hopefully poised to complete.

"That could be a problem," Elizabeth interjected, looking at me. I had to agree. The words *Tom* and *co-operate* would not usually find themselves side-by-side in a sentence.

"We can try though, can't we?" My gaze swung from one of them to the other and back again. "We've got to get him sorted out."

<u>How did Tom React when Refused Money?</u>

1. Accept this decision without question?
2. Threaten to smash up the house?
3. Steal some?
4. Threaten to wreck my car?
5. Think about getting a weekend job?
6. Inform me his is not going to school?
7. Try to break into someone's house?
8. Steal something that he can then sell?
9. Tell me that he will be beaten up unless he repays a debt?
10. Lose his coat and one shoe?
11. Threaten to 'stove' my face in?
12. Call me every derogatory name in his repertoire?

Over the course of July, all outcomes apart from 1 and 5 occurred.

E-mail to his Dad

July 2008 (14 years, 7 months)

Dear Peter and Elizabeth,

Sorry for doing this by email but the following needs to be said.
I have done everything in my power for Tom and now I think it is your turn. I freely admit I have failed; perhaps you can do a better job.
I can no longer cope with him and have got Alex's wellbeing to consider.
The situation is making me poorly and for these reasons, I would like us to swap roles: for him to live with you during the week and I will have him at weekends. I have no qualms about changing his school as I think, given his reputation where he is, it would be a positive move.
If you agree to my suggestion, I will also transfer all the child benefits over to you.
I am sorry to land this on you but this might be Tom's only hope of not ending up in care.
Can you please discuss this together and let me know your decision as soon as you can.

Sarah

PS If you don't take him then I really am putting him into care. I have had enough.

Days passed.

No reply.

The Child and Adolescent Mental Health Team

July 2008 (14 years, 7 months)

"There are people behind the screen, Tom," announced one of the two beaming women.

From the letter they had sent, I knew that one of them was a child psychologist and the other, a child psychiatrist. The smiling one looked fresh out of university; her older counterpart was probably somewhere in her forties. "They're listening to our conversation."

"Why would they want to do that?" Tom yawned as he lolled back in his chair.

"I know it must seem a bit strange," chuckled the other woman. "But it's so they can help us decide how to support your mum with things."

The 'screen' consisted of a window with a blind behind it. I wondered how many people it concealed and felt mildly defensive at the prospect of being 'judged' by unseen eyes.

The room we were in was less 'clinical' than on our previous visits, five years earlier. It had been carpeted and adorned with 'arty' pictures. Easy chairs had replaced stiff plastic ones. The 'medical' smell lingered though. As did the provision of a tissue box on the low table, that divided us all. It would be likely only me that would have a use for tissues, once we got going!

Tom remained slumped, repeatedly sketching a cartoon of SpongeBob Square Pants. "I'm not saying owt if a load of weirdo's are listening."

"They're not weirdo's, honestly." One of the women rose up and offered her arm to him. "Come on, I'll take you to meet them." As she led him behind the screen, I listened as several introductions were made. They returned moments later; all smiles.

Nervously, I waited for the women to proceed.

"Right," began the older one. "Firstly might I say how nice it is to meet you Tom, and mum. She nodded towards me. "We've been doing a little reading from a few years ago when you worked with Victoria Harris." Pausing, she smiled as she peered towards Tom. "Do you remember her Tom?"

He shook his head.

"He can barely remember what he ate for breakfast," I teased him. "Let alone someone he met five years ago!"

"I gather things have moved on a bit since then," she went on, "and according to your GP and Tom's school, you've been having a few more problems."

He shrugged his shoulders. My mouth opened in readiness to reply but the younger woman got there first.

"We *do* want you to be part of this process Tom." She spoke as though she was trying to load sincerity into her voice. "No meetings are going to happen without *you* being here. You're a big lad now and it's only fair you hear what's being discussed and let us know what's going on for you."

"Not a right lot." He scowled.

Smiling again at him, she continued. "We're going to be looking carefully at your relationship with your mum and seeing what improvements might be made." Turning to me, she asserted, "Sarah, I gather from the file that you had problems yourself as a child; particularly issues with your *own* mother. I think it's important that we begin by looking at that."

"I don't see how it's relevant." I felt irritated beyond words that they deemed my own background as a starting point.

"I'm not saying it is." Her face oozed with insincere sympathy. "Sometimes, though, it's inevitable that patterns from childhood are repeated. We need to explore that." Her eyes flickered from me to Tom and back again. "Perhaps we could arrange that discussion without Tom being present if that provides an easier environment for you to talk about such personal matters."

"I thought I was invited to all these meetings." Tom piped up.

"Well, maybe not the ones where we're talking to your mum about her stuff."

"It's all a waste of time anyway." Tom stretched his arms and legs out as he yawned. "There's nowt wrong with me."

"Oh yeah?" I challenged, wanting the focus to be shifted away from me. "So why do you carry on like you do?"

"Shut up Mum. You don't know what you're on about. As usual."

The two women blatantly watched our altercation; something about the way they stared at us and then at each other made me feel uneasy.

"We're going to be paying a lot of attention to the interaction between the two of you." The older woman looked at us in turn. "It will give us a lot of what we need at this stage."

"And what about the rest of the family? His dad? His stepdad? His stepmum? His brother? Surely their input is equally as important?"

"To start with we'll focus on the relationship just between the two of you. In these situations, it can provide the crux of the problem, and the starting point for rectification."

So that was it. The initial assessment. Clearly they were looking towards *me* for answers to Tom's problems. Blaming me. Already, I felt disillusioned. They didn't have a clue.

Good news!
A new house!
A new area!
A fresh start!

We are all praying that Tom does not spoil it!

The Youth Worker – Positive Activities for Young People)

What We Do

PAYP aims to prevent crime and reduce anti-social behaviour. PAYP staff have experience of working with individual children and young people aged 11—19 and their families. PAYP works in partnership with other professionals to access the needs of individual children and young people and develop individually tailored support packages aimed at preventing offending behaviour, supporting the transition from primary to secondary school, supporting children, young people and their families to build positive relationships and providing access to high quality opportunities to participate in positive activities.

Who We Work With

Vulnerable children and young people aged 11—19 who are at risk of becoming engaged in crime and anti-social behaviour. Schools, Social Services, YOT, Education Services, Police and other staff can refer individual children and young people to the PAYP Project.

<u>Tom's delinquent behaviour was rewarded with the following opportunities:</u>
- Days out at theme parks
- Football tickets
- Go-carting
- Cinema trips
- 10-pin bowling
- Quad biking
- Activity days
- Museum visits

<u>Quote from Alex</u>
"How come Tom is naughty but gets to do nice things?"

Answers on a postcard, please.

Playing With Fire 4 – Exclusion 6

September 2008 (14 years, 9 months)

"Is that Sarah?" It was Tom's head of year. Again. I knew the voice well and shuffled away from eavesdropping ears of other parents at Alex's sports day.

"It is."

"Do you want the good or the bad news?"

"I think I'll go for the good. There's not too much of that where Tom's concerned!"

"Well, he's eventually arrived at school. He got here at 10.25; but isn't in uniform and appears to be under the influence of something! But he's actually *here*!"

Groaning, I leaned against a wall. "That's the *good* news? I dread to think what the bad is!"

"I'm afraid we've just had to evacuate the entire school yet again. Tom set off the fire alarms."

"Oh for God's sake! How?" In exasperation, I raised my voice. Several people in my vicinity glanced over, enquiringly.

"By holding a lighter against the cctv camera in the boy's cloakroom. All the front of it melted, causing it to smoke and ………."

"Oh no! I'm so sorry!" I moved further away from the nosy mothers who were watching me intently and tried to lower my voice.

"Don't *you* be sorry! It's Tom who should be sorry. I'm well aware that he'll be delighted to be excluded from school. But there's nothing else we can do in the circumstances."

"How long?"

"Until the end of next week." The apology was unmistakeable within his voice. "The head's insisted."

"And the cost of the damage?" Reddening, I realised one or two eavesdroppers had heard my side of the conversation.

"I'll have to let you know."

The Electronic Tagging Device

After the burglary and criminal damage incident, he was in no further bother with the police that year. But we were still in and out of court.

As he was proving unable to comply with his reparation order; the courts kept adding further hours of unpaid work onto it. Furthermore, he was not attending appointments with the youth offending team. After four breaches, the court decided to impose the punishment of a forced home curfew.

Initially, I was relieved that I would know his whereabouts between 7 pm and 7 am for three months. This, however, quickly turned to despair! We were all pushed to breaking point for the duration, forced to be constantly in his company and at the mercy of his foul moods!

The security team came to install the tag around his ankle and equip our home with the necessary device to monitor his comings and goings. Inspecting his protruding tag, a sense of hopelessness enveloped me. *Was this what it had come to?* Tom, of course, tried every ploy he could conjure up to outsmart the tag:

1. Unplug unit from power source and blame mother.
2. Snip it off ankle and pretend it snapped as result of a trip on staircase.
3. Use butter to slide it off foot.
4. Stretch it over foot.

The security firm became regular visitors, not caring what hour of the night it was. His repeated breaches meant more court appearances. Swiftly, I learnt to take plenty of reading matter to wile away the endless hours in the public waiting area, surrounded by foul-mouthed, unrepentant adolescents. It was torture otherwise.

Brought Home by the Police 3

October 2008 (14 years, 10 months)

Fatigue was overtaking the battle with worry. I had stared so long into the darkness that my eyes were stinging. There was no sign of him, even though it was nearly 2 am. He would catch the bus back to our former area as he was struggling to acclimatise to the new neighbourhood.

By now, we were on first name terms with many members of the security team as he repeatedly breached his curfew order!

The 'bing-bong' of the doorbell and what sounded like a police radio jostled me into complete consciousness. I shot out of bed and down towards the front door. My initial panic at seeing a police hat through the window of the door was quelled by a familiar blond head beside it. I flung the door open.

"Where've you been?" I raked my hand through my hair. "I've been worried sick about you!"

"A bit of communication between the two of you might not go amiss in future," stated the stony-faced policeman as he nudged Tom towards me. "We're not a taxi service, neither are we responsible for getting your son home safely. You are." His finger wagged in my direction.

"We've only just moved here." I was aware of how feeble my argument must have sounded. "My son not coming home is not exactly out of character. It's not as if I can get hold of him either. He's sold his phone."

"Do you realise he rang 999 to get a lift? Obviously, he's fourteen and vulnerable, which is why we've brought him back on this occasion. If it happens again, he'll be done for wasting police time. And invoiced for the expense involved in taking advantage of police resources. Do you understand?"

"There won't be a next time," I stammered. "I'm sorry."*

*Sorry had to be the most-used word in my vocabulary. I was sick of saying it!

Reasons He Can No longer go to his Dad's House

1. Constant pilfering of other people's belongings
2. Stealing money out of money boxes and birthday cards.
3. Smoking cannabis in same bedroom as sleeping baby brother.
4. They don't want him there. (Wish I could exercise the same opinion!)
5. He can't be bothered going anyway.

Exclusion Number 7

(Another letter to add to my collection)

Dear Mrs Pearson

I am writing to inform you of my decision to exclude your son for a fixed period of four days. The exclusion begins on Friday 4th October and ends on Wednesday 9th October. This means that he will not be allowed in school for this period.

I realise that this exclusion may be upsetting but the decision has not been taken lightly. Thomas was removed from class this morning for displaying defiance and causing disruption. The supply teacher* who was taking his class was distressed after the incident. Furthermore, when he was sent to the isolation unit, he continued to ignore instructions. This amounts to a breakdown of discipline and will not be tolerated.

You also have the right to see Thomas's school record. Should you wish to do so, please notify me in writing. There may be a charge for photocopying.

The school has set work for Thomas during the period of his exclusion. Please ensure that the work set by school is completed and returned to us promptly for marking.

We expect him to be back in school on Wednesday 11th October at 08:50 am, where he will report to reception before completing one day in the Isolation Unit.

Yours sincerely

Head Teacher

*I later discovered that the supply teacher originated from Poland and had been upset by Tom drawing a Nazi swastika on the classroom floor and doing a 'Hitler style' salute whenever she tried to reprimand him.

Another Year; Another List of:

a. <u>Tom's thefts</u>

- money (from wallets, purses, money boxes, cards)
- 2 play station games belonging to Alex
- Alex's binoculars
- Elizabeth's ring, left to her in her aunt's will
- Numerous mobile phones
- X box games belonging to his dad
- DVDs
- 2 bikes on separate occasions
- Beer and wine from fridge

b. <u>Tom's breakages</u>

- Remote control
- Microwave
- His computer monitor
- His computer mouse
- His computer keyboard
- His computer hard drive
- His trainers, so he could get new ones
- Crockery
- Walls
- Glasses
- His bike, trashed in temper because it had a puncture
- Security camera and lap top at school
- Criminal damage to lift
- His portable DVD player

One Foot in the Door

Tom began attending the pupil referral unit, which was a bus ride away.

Although electronically tagged, he had still managed to acquaint himself with the local 'undesirables' in our new neighbourhood. The moment his curfew fell at seven in the evening, he would hang out of his bedroom window, conversing with them as they loitered on our driveway. The jerking of neighbouring curtains made me cringe and I begged him not to socialise in this way. My pleas, as always, fell on deaf ears.

One evening, as we watched TV, a pungent herby waft drifted into the house. I jumped up to investigate this all-too-familiar aroma. Tom's tagged foot held the front door ajar whilst the remainder of him smoked a joint on the other side. Wrenching the door open, I was horrified to see around twelve shadowy youths, all congregated on my driveway, passing several joints between them. Momentarily they paused their activity as they acknowledged my fury.

"Get away from my house! Now! The lot of you!"

Several of them sniggered. Hairs of rage prickled at the nape of my neck.

"Fuck off silly cow!"

"I'll call the police!" I shrieked, just wanting them anywhere but in front of my house.

"You're making a show of yourself mum!" Tom turned and hissed at me. "Sort yourself out!"

At that, I shoved him from the doorstep with all my might.

"You stupid fucking cow!" He squared up to me. "The tagging people'll be round now!"

"Get lost, all of you!" I stood in my doorway, hands on hips. "That includes you!" I gestured towards Tom.

Martin was now behind me. Pushing beyond me, he strode towards Tom.

"Get this sorted now, you little shit!" He grabbed him by the scruff of the neck. "We're not having this on our own doorstep!"

I threw Tom's coat and shoes at him before closing the door on the lot of them.

"You'd better watch your cars!" and "We'll be putting your fucking windows through!" reverberated in our ears through the door as Martin and I stared at each other, in absolute angst. Indeed, I lived in constant dread that they would carry out their threats.

Arrest Number 4, Another Court Appearance

"Well that's my evening ruined!" I replaced the receiver and exhaled deeply. "I've got to be the appropriate adult. He's been arrested again!" An eternal night at the police station loomed.

"What's he done this time?" Martin did not raise his eyes from the newspaper.

"The idiot has drawn graffiti all over a bus." Marching into the kitchen, I then began slamming pots into the dishwasher. "The woman on the phone says they've got him on cctv. So he'll definitely be done for it."

"You mean we will," Martin spoke smugly from his armchair.

As soon as I arrived at the station, I knew I would be in for a lengthy wait. The reception area was crammed. For nearly an hour, I had to stand before finally being escorted to the custody area. I nearly gagged at the stench of stale sweat which lingered in the air. Because of Tom's age it was necessary for me to be present whilst they formally 'booked him in.'

"We'll be with you in a few moments," growled the desk sergeant, not even glancing up from his paper shuffling.

Feeling insignificant and humiliated; I absorbed my now-not-so-unfamiliar surroundings. The 'admissions' board communicated that every cell was occupied. Silently, I berated him for getting arrested on a Friday. I scanned the board for his name. *Ah, yes. Cell Number Seven.* My gaze travelled around. There, outside cell number Seven, sat his lace-up trainers in case he was tempted to hang himself in the cell. The heat was stifling and I longed for the air outside. I had been stood for so long that I felt light-headed and was beginning to sway a bit.

"Do you mind if I sit while I wait? I don't feel good."

Mercifully one of the officers took pity on me, gave me a cup of water, and led me into the cooler interview room.

Several minutes later, Tom appeared in socks and paper trousers. (There had been a cord in his tracksuit bottoms.) Awkwardly, his eyes met mine.

"You idiot." That was about all I could muster up!

Absently, I listened as his rights were read. Next he was fingerprinted, photographed and swabbed. I observing these procedures then was sent away again. Meanwhile, Tom was led back to his cell.

"Please don't make me go back in there!" A couple of feet before the doorway, he brought himself to a halt.

"You should've thought about that before." The officer tried to shove Tom forwards.

"I can't stand it in there any more." Tom's imploring eyes sought mine. "Please don't make me."

"Look Tom. It's just for a while. Stop causing a fuss." The officer secured the heavy door behind him. Mournfully, I looked on, obviously powerless to intervene.

"If I give you my mobile number, can you let me know when you are ready to interview him/" I fished around in my bag to check I had my phone. "I'm going to read in my car. I can't stand it in the waiting area."

"You can see how busy we are." He watched as I scribbled my number onto a scrap of paper. "But we'll give you a call when we're ready."

Two hours went by before they summoned me back. By then I had devoured two magazines, a newspaper and half a novel. Tom looked desperate as he was brought back into the interview room.

"Can I go home after this?"

"Let's just wait and see, shall we?" The officer began unwrapping two tapes as he spoke to me. "Have you been an appropriate adult before?"

"I'm afraid so." I sat down, as directed and draped my cardigan over the back of my chair.

"Right you know the drill then. OK Tom," he announced briskly, I'm just going to go through your rights again, and then I'll check you understand them."

He began to ask a series of questions. *Does the bus belong to you? Do the seats you drew on belong to you? Were you intending to clean your graffiti off?*

"For the benefit of the tape I am showing the accused *exhibit a*," stated the officer, placing an item before us onto the graffiti daubed table.

As I surveyed this item, I struggled to contain my mirth. There, in a clear polythene bag, was a solitary permanent marker.

"Is this the implement you used to deface the bus?" he went on, oblivious to the laughter I was trying to quell. Luckily Tom was unaware of it too. Clearly, it was a serious situation but his line of questioning was so ridiculous that I was relieved to escape back to the sanctuary of my car. In the meantime, Tom was replaced in his cell whilst they decided what to do with him.

Three weeks later we were back in court. Happily this time, *he* was punished and given fifteen hours of reparation. Cleaning buses!

Family Life

Whilst at court, I also withdrew permission for the tagging equipment to remain in our house. We were living on a knife's edge, waiting for him to surface at seven each evening and enduring the visit of the security firm when he *didn't* return.

Twice, I had been back in court as a result of 'the three strikes and you're out' system. Basically, Tom had got wise to the fact that it was only on his *third* non-appearance, that he would be hauled back to court. There the magistrate would bestow a 'stern reprimand,' and Tom could return to 'strike one' again.

It had been 'hell on earth' having him among us from seven each evening; the whole atmosphere would descend as soon as he walked in. Either he would be stoned or in a mood so foul, (sometimes both), that we would feel like running for cover.

The neighbours now shunned us all; evidently they were judging our entire family by the endless presence of hoods, gathered like ghouls, at the front of my house. Even the neighbours next door no longer permitted their daughter to play with Alex in our house.

Tom rejoiced at the tag's removal.

"Don't think it means you can do whatever you want," I warned, shaking my finger at him. If you're not home by half past ten, the door will be locked from now on."

It was impossible to adhere to this, when at two, three or four o'clock in the morning, he would beat on the door and repeatedly ring the bell until I responded. Really, he only came home to eat and sleep. Oh, and to thieve and bully me for money.

"What am I supposed to do with an effing fiver!" He snatched at a note I had left on the kitchen worktop.

"It's all I've got."

"You're a lying bitch! Show me your purse."

"I'll do no such thing!" I thrust the note back into my bag. "And how dare you speak to me like that!"

Cowering in my room, I listened as he slammed around. Then, with one final bang of the door, I heaved a sigh of relief at the realisation he had gone out. Returning downstairs, I began to make a camomile tea to soothe my fractured nerves.

"Mummy, two of my best games have gone?" Alex appeared in the kitchen doorway, worry etched across his face.

"Gone?" My heart plummeted, innately suspecting where they would have gone. "Are you sure?"

"I left them next to my play station." He pointed back up the stairs. "They were there before. *Little Big Planet* and *Fifa 09.*"

Trailing him up to his room, I hoped to be able to find them myself. The cost of them had exceeded sixty pounds that Christmas. As I had feared, my search proved fruitless.

"Oh well. I guess they've gone then." Alex slumped miserably onto his bed. "It probably serves me right for not hiding them better."

I wanted to weep for him. All he possessed that was saleable, was at Tom's mercy. It had been a long time since he had given up attempting to save in his piggy bank.

Tom startled me that evening when he lurched through the door before midnight. This was virtually unheard of on a Friday evening! I was poised to 'let rip' about Alex's missing games but my attention was diverted to the state he was in.

"Oh my God! What's happened to you?" Spotting his swollen aw, I gasped. Then I noticed that he was clutching his leg. His torn tracksuit bottoms laid bare an angry gash. "You're going to need stitches!" I was horrified.

"It's nowt Mum. Stop panicking. I got into a fight that's all. The cut's not as bad as it looks." He flinched as I inspected it. "I'm ore bothered about me trackies. Can you sew em?"

Changing Stories

"Who were you fighting with?" By the next day his leg had already begun to heal and thankfully did not seem to need stitching after all.

"This lad." He winced as I peeled the dressing further back. "No one you know."

"What was it about?" I dabbed at the wound with antiseptic.

"Look Mum. Leave it." He tried to pull his leg away. "I don't wanna talk about it. Alright?"

"Well I do." Gently yanking the leg back towards me, I began to apply the fresh dressing.

"Ok, ok. I'll tell you what happened. Me mates were carrying on over who'd paid for what with a crate of beer and it got out of hand. I tried to break it up. A bottle got trashed and a piece of glass bounced up and cut into me leg."

"Don't insult my intelligence Tom. That's impossible. A piece of glass bouncing up from the ground would not cause that much damage." From a roll, I snipped a length of bandage to wrap around his leg.

"Don't believe me then. Do I look bothered?"

"Have you heard about the woman attacked at the bus station?" I could not meet his eyes.

"Yeah, what about it?" His voice hardened.

"What do *you* know about it?"

"Nowt really. Didn't see much of it. Was round the corner having a smoke. What you accusing me of now?"

"But you were there?"

"It wasn't me. Honest Mum." Searching his face, I was convinced I could detect panic within it. "In fact I stopped with her till the ambulance got there."

"It says in the paper that the police got there first." I pointed to where the paper lay on the coffee table.

"It's in the paper?" Snatched it up, he flicked through the pages for the article.

"Of course it is. She was badly hurt." I tried to keep my voice steady as I trembled inside. *God he was there!*

"Not by me, she wasn't." Having located the article, he shook the paper out in front of him. "I tried to help her get up off the floor."

"Was it your mates who did it?"

"No. Well, kind of. Some of em. Not the ones that were hurting her though."

"Was that where you injured your leg?" Having re-bandaged his wound, I secured it with elastoplast.

"I've already told you what happened. Someone chucked a bottle and it cut through me trackies."

"Who threw it then?"

"I dunno!" He slapped the newspaper back onto the table. "Will you stop going on! You're blagging my head?"

"A moment ago you told me it was your mate who smashed the bottle." I remained on my knees upon the floor, seemingly begging for his honesty.

Howling with rage, he stormed out. I sat, absently studying the sun reflecting back from the living room table. My daffodils looked well in the window.

Breathing slowly, in through the nose and out through the mouth, like I had learned at yoga, I tried to calm myself down.

My conscience would not have let me rest if I had not taken action. It was a compulsion. I rang the local police station and informed them about Tom's injury and the fact that he had admitted to being within the vicinity of the attack.

Arrest Number 5

It took them two days to arrest him. In the meantime, I could barely look at him. I was convinced he had been instrumental in the violent attack of this poor woman.

"It'll be some time before we get round to interviewing him," advised the arresting officer as he cuffed him. "We've another two of them to pick up yet."

Later that evening I got a call to say they were ready for me. Again I waited in the furnace of the custody area, scanning for trainers which would verify which cell he was in. Not that it made much difference to anything that was going on.

"We've had a few problems with him." The desk sergeant surveyed me coolly from behind the towering, green desk. Below his sweat-soaked receding head, waded definite disapproval in his eyes. "Evidently he doesn't appreciate being locked up. He's demonstrated this by head butting the wall. Claims he's trying to knock himself out."

"Is he OK?" Panic soared in me like bile. Memories of him head banging in his bedroom as a toddler resurfaced. "Have you checked on him?"

"Yep. Just a sore head. The first aider's been keeping an eye. He's not done himself any favours mind. We'll be interviewing him last. After his accomplices."

Groaning inwardly, I retreated to the refuge of my car to read. Not that I could concentrate on anything at that moment.

Dusk was descending, projecting a shadow over the formidable police station. The 'windows' of the cells were visible, just above ground level. They were dimly lit, compared to the rest of the windows. Contained behind one of them, I imagined my son as I tried to bury the displaced guilt that was consuming me.

After what seemed like an eternity, they were finally ready to interview. Tom's head was raw with injury as they escorted him to the green desk to read out the charge.

I shook my head at him. "What the hell possessed you to do that to yourself?"

He refused a solicitor. "I'm not waiting for one of them to get here. I just want to get on with it."

Before commencing the interview, they photographed the injury on his leg. It did not dawn on him to question this; if he had, my initial telephone call to the police might have come to his attention.

In his interview, he gave the same story he had told me, about having been there, helping the woman, and waiting with her for the ambulance.

"And you were present whilst she was being beaten?"

"I was standing nearby." His face twitched as he strove to maintain eye contact with his questioner.

"You could see what was happening? And you didn't think to help her?" He frowned at Tom.

"I did help her. After they had stopped."

"Who's they?"

"I dunno." Nervously, he shrugged.

"We've got the whole thing on cctv. Are you aware of that?" The officers eyes widened as he studied Tom for a reaction.

"No."

"So when we examine it, we'll see you, just *watching*? Then *helping*? We won't see you contributing to her injuries?"

"No." Then suddenly Tom's composure crumbled. "I don't care whether you believe me or not!" His half-broken voice rasped around the poky room. "I didn't hurt no-one!"

Eventually, he was released on police bail, pending further enquiries. We were to return the following week.

Over the next few days it felt like a hurricane cloud was nestling above me. I hardly told anyone what was going on. The shame enveloped me like an ill-fitting cardigan. The guilt I was experiencing towards the victim was palpable.

The day came when I was to accompany him to answer his bail. I felt jubilant that I managed to get him back to the station at the required time. He had put up quite a fight.

"I'm not getting done for summat I've not done!" He seemed agitated as he travelled in the passenger seat.

"If that's true then you've nothing to worry about." Clenching the steering wheel, I prayed he was telling the truth, but I could not help suspecting the worst.

"But what if someone who isn't me, looks like me on the cameras?"

"Tom, I don't know. We'll see when we get there." By now, I was desperate to get it over with.

"I'm not going in no cell," he announced as we parked in the station car park. "I'll head-butt the copper this time if he thinks he's putting me in there."

"Don't be ridiculous." Locking the car, I sighed as we headed towards the sliding entrance door.

"I will." He dragged himself along behind me. "Just watch me."

They did lock him back up. But he went into the cell like a lamb, despite his previous bravado. The officer closed the heavy cell door and there was a loud clunk as he turned the key. I surveyed Tom's trainers in dismay.

"At least I know where he is tonight," I joked, fishing in my bag for my book whilst trying to find light in the darkness of the situation.

"Take a seat in the waiting area love," the desk sergeant nodded from behind the desk. "We'll try not to keep you too long."

Again, I slayed the dawdling time by trying to read. Before long, my backside was deadened from being perched on the chilly, solid metal of the waiting room bench. My head ached in the glare of the blazing fluorescent strip-lights. The automatic entrance doors responded to every passing bird or whisper of a breeze and continually startled me.

Occasionally someone would come in. They would state their business in hushed tones through the intercom and I would eavesdrop, nosily. One man tried making conversation with me. He stunk of stale drink and I wished he would leave me alone with my book and my thoughts. Finally, a policeman's voice sliced into my boredom.

"Can I have a word?" Snapping my book shut, I dutifully followed him into a side room.

"We're going to have to let him go." He shook his head. "We've not enough evidence to charge him."

"But the cctv....."

"It's too grainy. They all look the same. They're dressed almost identically. The CPS won't let us charge any one unless we've got something a lot more than what we've got."

"Do you not recognise anyone on the cctv?"

He shook his head again sadly. "Unless any of them admit anything, we've got nothing."

"They've got away with it. I don't believe it. That poor woman!"

Tom was euphoric upon leaving the police station. Me, I felt like slapping him.

Brought Back by the Police 4

"We discovered him in an inebriated state and vomiting in the middle of town," announced the policeman, ripping back the sliding door of the police van. Tom slopped, like custard skin, onto the pavement. "So we're returning him to you." Hauling him to his feet, he led him towards me. "Miraculously, he remembered where he lived! May I suggest that you get him inside and put him to bed?"

"Look at the state of you! You're a bloody disgrace!" Yanking him inside, I gagged at the stench of regurgitated lager that clung to him.

The policeman turned on his heel, before retreating back towards his van, shaking his head all the time as he proceeded.

Brought Back By The Police 5

It was exactly a week later when a police van drew up outside yet again. Its formidable form emitted a shadow over the house.

Oh for God's sake! What now? I scuttled to respond to the door.

"Is this your son?" The policeman surveyed me as though I were an insect.

"I'm afraid so."

"The next time we find him in this state, we'll lock him up for the night. Is that clear?"

"Lock him up now if you want." I suddenly felt defiant.

"We shouldn't have to. You should be keeping him under control." His finger wagged in my direction.

"I'm trying to. You've no idea what it's like!" My hand flew to my forehead as I tried to brush my anxiety away. "He's out of windows if we try to keep him in!"

"Well, we've better things to be doing with our resources than to be fishing reprobates like your son off the streets!" Muttering still, he turned and retreated to his van.

Tom had slithered past me and put himself to his bed. Silently, I fumed as I ascended the stairs and placed a bucket beside him. Backing away from him, I was grateful to reach the oxygenated landing where I could take a breath of normal smelling air before I passed out!

On his Own Doorstep 1

We had lived on the new housing estate for several months. Only a fraction of the other houses were occupied. Typically the inhabited homes were all within hearing and seeing distance from ours so Tom's conduct had been witnessed in full glory.

The site manager had made us aware that prospective buyers were put off by the youths hanging around. Before long their presence took a downward turn.

"Bloody hell!" exclaimed Martin, abruptly pausing and emitting a slow whistle. We were walking the dog in the street running perpendicular from our house, therefore it was out of our view usually.

Together, our eyes wandered from one house to the next and the next. The yet-to-be-loved homes drooped sadly in the early spring sunshine. Lanterns and drainpipes had been ripped from walls. There were two smashed windows and a warped garage door.

"Oh no! This will cost a fortune to put right!" A bin cupboard door in one of the porches swayed on one hinge instead of three and someone had lit a fire inside. A bowed garage door was peppered with scorch marks; as though somebody had a burning object against it. Litter was strewn everywhere. Splodges of mud remained from where 'mud bombs' had pelted the houses. Then I noticed the graffiti adorning the walls. The same signature had been repeated over and over. As had numerous sketchings of SpongeBob Squarepants!

"Have a look at this Martin!" My heart thudded as reality dawned.

"Yep, it's definitely him. It's the same signature that he's drawn all across his bedroom wall. He calls it his 'tag.'" Pausing, he surveyed me intently, as though expecting a reaction.

"Talk about doing the proverbial on your own doorstep."

"It's this kind of thing that could get us kicked out of the house." Yanking hold of the dog's lead, we began to walk away. "Somehow we've got to stop them!"

Later that evening, as we relaxed in the garden, the usual din erupted outside, indicating that once again, the teenagers had landed! There was a restricted view of the 'action' available from the landing window. Martin sped upstairs, tailed by Alex and I.

"They're at it again!" observed Martin, leaning onto the windowsill. "There's a few of them!"

"Is Tom with them?"

"I can't see him."

There was a deafening bang before something smashed.

"I think you should ring the police Mummy!" Alex looked concerned as he stood on tiptoes, trying to see.

"If you come now you'll catch them all in action." I informed the operator as I paced the room. "They must be costing the building company a fortune!"*

For several minutes we waited, expecting a police van to screech up and sling them all in the back. Instead, after about half an hour, a lone police officer came trundling down the street on a cycle.

My laugh was hollow as I ventured outside.

The teenagers quickly disbanded as the officer pointed his bike in their direction.

"If the information I gave had been acted on properly;" I called out; "you would've caught them all."

"I know," he conceded, scratched under his cycle helmet. "I just go where I'm sent.

*As a result of the above, the building company employed a 'security guard' to patrol the housing estate each night. To be honest, he spent most of his shift 'holed up' in one of the empty apartments. Most of the occupants harboured reservations about what this middle-aged, obese, lone man in a security uniform would be able to achieve against the might of the local hoods anyway.

Magistrates Warnings

As a result of Tom's frequent court order breaches, I became a 'regular, at court. Having my handbag checked and being searched using a handheld body scanner became second nature. It grew increasingly amusing to listen to the various warnings and reprimands given to him:

"If you return to this court, you'd better bring your toothbrush!"
"You can be assured that I'll be dealing with you personally in future!"
"If I see you in this court again, you'll be leaving by this door, not from that one!"
"If you end up back here, you might as well bring your pyjamas!"
"You will be finding out just how hard life is inside a young offender's institution if you are brought before me again!"
"Any more breaches and we'll have a prison van waiting for you!"
"I've made a note on your file. If I see you again, your mother will be getting a nice long break from you!"
"You'll be needing to bring your slippers if you return to this court!"

I wanted to laugh out loud each time I heard one of these 'harsh' warnings being issued. Tomwould nod earnestly as though he actually took them seriously.

Full Circle

This chapter has been given this title because in terms of sleep, we went right back to the beginning. Every night. If we were not woken by revving engines or stones being hurled up at Tom's window, we were woken by Tom himself. It would then take forever to get back to sleep. I would lie awake, awaiting further interruption, continually turning the problems around in my mind.

One night I was alarmed to hear voices on our landing. Sitting bolt upright, I froze.

"There's someone in the house!" I hissed at Martin, elbowing him. "Didn't you lock the door?"

"I left it unlocked for Tom. I'm sick of being woken at all hours." There was a rap on our door. Martin leapt out of bed.

"What the hell do you think you're doing?" Two teenagers, slightly younger than Tom, cowered before him.

"Tom's got my bag," stammered one, backing away. "He nicked it."

"So you just stroll into my house?"

"I need the bag."

"Get out of here now, before I physically throw you out!" He started towards the boys who sprinted down the stairs and away into the darkness.

Tom stayed out all night. I lay awake, staring into the blackness; consumed with anxiety about the 'bag situation,' but also devoured by my usual fear for Tom's whereabouts. Eventually, I must have drifted off as I was abruptly awoken to a thumping at the front door. In my foggy haze, I tugged on my dressing gown and tried to peer inconspicuously through the blinds. Whoever was at the door was out of my vision, either concealed by the porch or perhaps trying round the rear of the house. I prayed it was Tom.

I was worn out with never having any idea of who he was with or what he was up to. His last mobile phone had lasted eleven days before he had sold it, so it wasn't as if I could even contact him. Reaching for the door handle, I noticed the bedroom clock. *6.20.*

"Great, I might as well get up." There would be no point trying to go back to sleep now.

The banging became more urgent and jostled me into a swift descent down the stairs. Through the small windows at the top of the door, I saw two heads, two hats, two police officers! In horror, I realised, that at 6.20 am, this was no social call. It *must* be bad news. Maybe the unspeakable dread I lived and stayed awake with each night had been realised. *Tom!* Trembling, I tried to turn the key. Each of my heartbeats was lurching upwards. The police must have sensed my terror as they surveyed me. The female officer smiled.

"It's OK. He's in custody."

Heaving a sigh of relief, I leaned against the doorframe. "Thank God. For a moment......"

"I know. Don't worry." She stretched her arm out towards me. "Can we come in?"

Widening the door, I invited their entry. At least at this hour, net curtains would not be twitching. There won't be many mothers who would feel such intense relief at the news of an incarcerated son, but the alternatives were beyond contemplation.

"What's he done this time?"

"Possession with intent to supply," stated the male officer, matter-of-fact.

"Oh no!" I plunged down onto a chair.

"We caught him coasting around in a car with two others at around three this morning."

A car! Now I was even more worried. I had heard about loads of tragic accidents that occur in the night by teenagers who had got hold of cars!

"We discovered over £200 in cash, in the car, weighing scales and a substantial quantity of cannabis."

"If you've had him since three, how come you've only just let me know?" I glanced at the clock again.

"We need to search your house." The policewoman's eyes skimmed the room. "To have informed you of his arrest might have given you opportunity to conceal or move things."

"I wouldn't have done that."

"I'm not suggesting you would. But some parents might."

"You won't find anything, you know. Do I look like the sort of person who would have anything to do with drugs?" Although who knows what I looked like at that hour of the morning!

I felt mildly offended as she plucked two pairs of rubber gloves from her pocket What did she expect to be contaminated with?

"Can I wake my husband?" Springing from the chair, I tightened the cord of my dressing gown. "I think he'll get a bit of a shock if two police officers burst into the bedroom!"

"OK, we'll start searching down here first." She offered a pair of the gloves to her colleague.

Martin had already emerged from the bed and was swiftly dressing.

"It's just one thing after another.

"Is it OK if we come up?" the policewoman startled us.

They searched Tom's room quickly. Other than his clothes, his possessions were of meagre proportions, which made me desperately sad when I allowed myself to consider it. Most of what he had owned had been sold to fund his cannabis addiction.

They moved towards Alex's door.

"You don't have to ransack my seven-year-old's room surely?" They looked at each other.

"I'm afraid we're obliged to search the entire house." The policeman pushed his door ajar.

"You won't find anything in there." Alex's dark hair was poking out from under his duvet. Whilst he slept, he always burrowed right under it. "He's still asleep for God's sake!"

Thankfully they agreed to leave his room alone. Back downstairs we needed to complete paperwork in view of the fact that they had searched our home but had not seized anything.

"What's your occupation," The policewoman waited, her pen poised.

"Teacher." My voice was barely audible.

"You're a teacher?" she shrieked. "And you can't even control your own son?"

I stared at my feet, feeling as low as them.

"Hey, that's not fair," It was comforting that Martin had jumped to my defence. "You don't know the background. You're forming opinions without the knowledge of what we've been through with him."

Without offering an apology, she persisted with her form, but mercifully passed no further judgement. Silently though, I fumed. I was only too aware that she had voiced what most people probably thought. *No, I couldn't control him.* I could have scoured every corner of the country and been lucky to find anybody who could.*

*I subsequently spent nearly four hours at the police station whilst he and his two accomplices were interviewed and re-interviewed. The police had the cheek to request that I act as appropriate adult to one of other people! Apparently their own parent had refused to attend! In the end all three denied any knowledge of the cannabis, cash or scales, each blaming one of the others!

The CPS concluded the crime could not be reliably pinned on any one individual; therefore they were all released without charge. Me, I'd have charged the bloody lot of them!

I Could Have Papered The Wall With These

Teaching and Learning Centre
Easton Drive
Yorkshire
YD16 6NE

9th July 2009

Dear Parent/Carer,

Re: Tom Clifford

I am writing to inform you of my decision to exclude Tom for a fixed period of one afternoon.

This means that he will not be allowed in school for this period. The exclusion is for one afternoon, 9th July 2009.

I realise that this exclusion may be upsetting for you and your family, but the decision to exclude Tom has not been taken lightly. Tom has been excluded for this fixed period because he absconded from the centre and is suspected of being under the influence of an illegal substance.

You have the right to make representations to the education authority about this decision. These representations will be considered by Inclusion Services.

If you think this exclusion related to a disability your child has, and you think disability discrimination has occurred, you may raise this issue with the governing body.

You also have a right to see of copy of Tom's school record. Due to confidentiality restrictions, you will need to notify me in writing if you wish to be supplied with a copy. There may be a charge for photocopying.

Tom's exclusion expires on Thursday 9th July 2009 and we expect him to be back in school on Friday 10th July 2009. Should you have any queries, please contact me.

Yours sincerely
Head of Centre

Parents Evening

I braced myself as I pressed the intercom at the pupil referral unit. Unlike mainstream secondary schools, the exits were kept locked. Not that this ever deterred Tom. Regular phone calls kept me up to speed with his escapes. Through windows, over walls; once he'd had enough, he was out of there. Not that he was learning a great deal in any case. Apart from where to score cannabis and who in the unit might join him in smoking it. Often, he was ejected from the centre for being 'under the influence' therefore 'unteachable.' (See letter above!)

It was debatable how much teaching went on anyway. There was never a single book or worksheet that accompanied him home. I welcomed the opportunity to discover if he had actually made any progress throughout his time there.

"He's gifted at art," affirmed his 'key-worker,' Lynn, who spoke in a throaty voice and reeked of cigarettes, even though she sat at the other side of the table from me. "We think he's a potential candidate for art college."

"Well, that's something." I waited for the 'but.' If Tom had purpose; ambition........anything, then maybe he would be diverted from his current road of destruction. It was wonderful to hear something positive, a chink of hope.

The class sizes in the centre were miniscule compared to 'normal' classes; a maximum of eight teenagers occupied each one. It was to be hoped that the staff would get well acquainted with the kids they were teaching.

"But he'd have to get off the cannabis," she continued, dragging me back down to earth. "He's stoned nearly every day. There's no way he can concentrate or retain anything in that state."

"The only person who can get Tom to stop smoking cannabis is *Tom*. All kinds of drug interventions have already been attempted by his last school *and* by the youth offending team. He's got to *want* to stop."

"How much money do you give him?" *Great they are blaming me, as usual.* The jowls in her neck wobbled as she tipped her head in anticipation of my reply.

"The bare minimum." I looked straight into her face. "But I suspect even his lunch money goes on weed."

"Have you tried giving him sandwiches?"

"Of course I have." Leaning forward, I clasped my hands together. "He won't even put them in his bag. Anyway, if I don't give him any money at all, he's unbearable *and* more likely to steal stuff from home."

For a moment she sat, frowning as though she was rehearsing her reply carefully. "We should discuss that 'unbearable' side you mention. Whenever he's *not* stoned, he's usually short tempered. In fact, we've had a few incidences of him swearing at other pupils or staff."

"I can imagine. I know exactly what he's like." I glanced down at the sheet of notes she had in front of her. "Anyway, other than artwork, how's he getting on with his other lessons?"

"Well, he's got interesting ideas but the attention span of a flea." She chuckled slightly but it was not a genuine laugh. "Even when we do manage to interest him, it's short lived. So he disrupts the others whose concentration skills are no better than his."

"But you're coping with him aren't you?" Without waiting for an answer, I continued. "It's just that he's had dreadful problems in his schools before." *That was an understatement!*

"He's not one of our *better* pupils." She looked apologetic. "But we've encountered worse, don't worry! If he can kick the weed, I think he'd stand a fighting chance in life."

"I've begged, lectured, threatened and argued with him over it. It's out of my hands." I displayed the inside of my palms as if to enforce my point. "It's an informed choice. He's well aware of the dangers in smoking it; I've made sure of that. Base 10, you know, the drugs information service, have done too, and his youth offending team drugs worker."

"Hmmmm. Right, well, if that's the case, there does not seem much more we can do on that front." She looked thoughtful. "Not until the decision to sort the drugs problem comes from within him. Anyway, moving on from that…… I'm afraid there've been several complaints about him urinating outside." Pausing, she clearly expected a reaction of outrage from me. "Obviously, at his age, it's unacceptable." As she pursed her lips, the lines around them became more prominent. "The girls and female staff within the centre should not have to bear witness to it!"

"He's been doing it since babyhood!" Leaning back on my chair, I clasped my hands behind my head. "It's happened at every school he's ever been to! I'm not sure if he's trying to shock people or just can't be bothered finding a toilet." I glanced out of the window, noticing the metal fencing surrounding the building. "God only knows why he still does it now!"

"If you could have a word………"

"For what good it'll do." I raised my eyes to the yellowing ceiling.

The classroom was barren. The furniture might have been cast out by a mainstream school and the walls were crying out for displays that might stimulate enthusiasm. Later, as I ventured towards the exit, I noticed the walls of the disinfected corridors were just as devoid of any effort. Free rein had been granted for pupils at the centre to unleash their creativity at graffiti 'art' but there was no evidence of any learning or any link to the curriculum to which they should have been entitled.

The Child and Adolescent Mental Health Service (again)

My first encounter with this service, back when Tom was eleven, had been constructive. Although there had been no flick of a magic wand or medication offered; I had felt as though Victoria, the child psychiatrist, was thorough and non-judgmental.

At the time, the suggestions and advice she had offered had been a Godsend. The fact that she had diagnosed something, albeit Conduct Disorder instead of ADHD; had added weight to my claims that Tom's condition was beyond the realms of any errors I might have made as a parent.

Unfortunately, I was not as lucky with the 'experts' that now confronted us at each appointment. When I say 'us,' I mean 'me.' And when I say 'confronted,' I mean 'besieged.'

"Do you not think your negative attitude is making things worse?" one of them challenged me. I seethed silently, knowing that Tom would be saving up these comments to fire back at me later.

"*You'd* be negative if you had to live with him." We glared at each other, the echoes of his usual attitude on the journey over still lingering.

"But surely in front of him." the younger woman, the 'psychologist' was speaking, "a positive manner would be more beneficial."

"It was *you* that suggested Tom should be present for all these meetings." My reply carried an air of rebellion. "There's no point in me lying in front of him, is there? I need to tell it like it is."

"Yes, and we'll stand by that, for now anyway." Emptily, she smiled at me. "He should be here, to have his say. However we're concerned that it won't be doing his self esteem any good, hearing his own mother being so pessimistic about him." The other woman nodded her agreement.

"It's not doing *my* self esteem any favours being sworn at and insulted every day."

"We must remember who's the adult in all this." I shrank under the older woman's admonishing stare.

Tom lolled, laid back and calm in his chair. As always he sketched SpongeBob Square Pants repeatedly as we conversed. It was a nightmare persuading him to these appointments, requiring excessive amounts of bribery and coercion. I wished they had cameras in their waiting rooms. Especially that morning. They would have been able to witness the full might of his nasty tongue. Of course, he would swiftly switch from hostility towards me as we waited, to being all sweetness and flowers in front of these two women.

"I try to say sorry but *she* won't let me." I swear he was batting his eyes at them. Peering at him incredulously, I listened to a sample from his stock of 'one-liners' reserved for occasions such as this:

"She thinks more of my brother, Alex, than me."
"I'm going to get my head down and do well at school."
"I hardly smoke any cannabis now. People who do are stupid."
"I'm going into the army when I leave school."
"I'm going to work hard and prove my mum wrong."

The women intermittently smiled and nodded at his repertoire that I had been subjected to already on numerous occasions. It was frequently 'trotted' out, in an effort to yank the wool over the eyes of people in authority.

In this case, I was mildly amused to notice that the younger woman and Tom almost *flirted* with each other throughout our appointments. Both the psychologist and psychiatrist were seemingly viewing me with an air of dislike. There was no interest from them in respect of Tom's latest exploits and misdemeanours; they wanted to talk about the past, and only the past. It was exasperating.

It was the norm that half way through the appointment; Tom and I were split, as were the 'experts.' They would converse separately with either Tom or me.

"Anne and I have conferred and we believe that history is unfortunately repeating itself," the psychologist stipulated after the 'split' at that particular meeting. "You suffered so harshly being rejected in your teens by your own mother, that you're now allowing yourself to do the same thing to *your* son." Shifting uncomfortably, I felt myself being scrutinised, like a specimen beneath a microscope. "How do you feel about that?"

"It's a load of absolute rubbish!" Inwardly, I felt myself trembling as I leaned forward in my chair to quell it. "I only wish Tom had been 'blessed' with *my* mother, he would've been long gone! She couldn't have coped with a fraction of what I've had to!"

"You must admit you're in danger of rejecting him." Her tone was calm and level. I wondered how she could take such a prejudiced view from only seeing us a handful of times.

"You're wrong." I sat back again, and glared at her with challenge in my eyes. "It's because of my own background that I've persevered for so long. My role as a mother is something I treat *very* seriously. Why else would I keep trying to get help for him?"

"We don't see that there's any underlying medical condition that he needs *help* with." Her eyes conveyed her unspoken words: *I'm the expert here!*

My heart plummeted with a thud. *What a waste of time!* "But you're basing your opinions on limited time spent with us in an environment that's not even natural."

"Actually, we're basing our *judgement* on the interaction between the two of you that we've witnessed. As well as the previous reports we've read." She flicked at the pages of her file as it rested on her knee. "Even an educational psychologist previously thought that your relationship with Tom indicated an attachment disorder. And he was only nine then."

I snorted incredulously. "He observed him at school for an hour. How can he seriously make an informed judgement in that time?"

"Nevertheless," she skirted around the question as she pursued her argument. "I feel that future appointments would be better spent addressing your own mother's treatment and rejection of you, and how you're going to prevent your relationship with Tom from further deterioration."

"If he stopped taking drugs, being abusive and getting arrested; that might be a start." Uncrossing my legs, I sat up straight.

"But it's *you* who has to take responsibility for how he's turned out." As she raised her voice, she flung her hands up in the air. "It's you who brought him up."

"Not to take drugs and break the law! Listen, we're getting nowhere." Hauling my handbag from the floor, I dumped it onto my knee. "If you think I am going to rake up my childhood in front of you, you're mistaken."

"I understand it could be painful for you." Her voice was calmer now.

"It's not even relevant." I fished around in my bag for my keys. "Addressing Tom's issues is what matters."

"We're going to offer a specialist counsellor for him to meet with fortnightly. He can get things off his chest and perhaps discuss his drugs issues. But in the case of yourself; we can't force you to engage with help if you don't feel able to."

"I don't *need* help!" Steam was possibly starting to emit through my ears as I jumped to my feet! "Not personally anyway! I need help with *Tom!*"

Her face was flushed, though probably not as much as mine. I felt utterly failed. Blamed and judged.

"I just hope one day you're not reading about something he's done in the papers." I strode to the door." Because the way things are at the moment, anything's possible in the future! Tell him I'll be waiting in the car!"

The Weekly News

Spate of Late Night Shop Break-ins

Police suspect local Youths

Police and local traders were today appealing for help in finding what they believe to be youths, who are responsible for at least four break-ins at four shops within the last week. The latest, which took place in the early hours of yesterday morning, was captured on cctv both inside and outside the shop.

It is believed the thefts are linked; they have all been targeted within a mile radius of each other and have all suffered similar losses; cigarettes, large quantities of alcohol and confectionary.

If any member of the public has information which may lead police towards the culprits, they are asked to contact the local police station or ring Crimestoppers, in complete confidence on 0800 555111.

Arrest Number 7

"Come on Tom!" Jangling my keys, I hollered up the stairs for the third time. "We've got to be at the dentist in twenty minutes. "Get your teeth cleaned *now!* I'll wait for you in the car."

Eventually, he emerged, looking as though he had been dug up from somewhere!

"You should get yourself home at a reasonable hour," I remarked, ushering him out of the door so I could lock it. "You need your sleep you know, instead of rolling in after four in the morning. And I need mine." My voice was lifting as I ranted. "God knows what you're doing until that time anyway." It was more of a question than a statement.

"Stop chatting shit Mum." He closed his eyes. "My head can't take it today."

We passed the local shop which was being boarded up. Two of the windows had been smashed in. A police car crouched outside. I glanced at Tom who appeared to be grinning to himself.

"What's going on around here?" I exclaimed, suddenly recalling the newspaper article. "That's the fourth shop in a week to have been broken into. It must be the same......"

Stealing a sideward's glance at Tom, reality dawned. "I hope none of it's to do with you, because if the police were to ask, I'd have to say I didn't know where you were last night, well not until four in the morning anyway."

"Why d' you always have to think the worst of me?" His voice was feeble as he tried to load anger into it. "It's got fuck all to do with me!"

"Stop swearing at me!" I slammed the palm of my hand against the steering wheel. "What gives you the right to swear at me? You'll get out of this car and walk in a minute."

"I didn't want to go to the bloody dentist anyway." He took a sip of water from the bottle he was carrying.

When we arrived, he shot to the toilet. The waiting room and reception area echoed with the sounds of him retching and vomiting. Everyone's eyes bored into me as though I had poisoned him. I squirmed in my seat.

"You'll have to ask him to wait outside," ordered the receptionist, unable to mask the revolt on her face. "Obviously the dentist can't see him in that state."

"What's the matter with you?" I hissed as I led him out.

"Too much to drink, that's all." Groaning, he resumed his retching in the car park. Swiftly, I abandoned him, anxious not to watch or hear him!

For the rest of that day he slept. Until we received a loud banging at the door. It sounded like the police. And guess what? It was!

"Tom Clifford," barked the policeman. His female colleague stood demurely at his side.

"He's asleep." I groaned inwardly at the thought of having to cancel that evening's plans to be his appropriate adult, yet again.

"We need to speak to him in connection with local shop burglaries," stated the policewoman, stepping towards me. "You'll have to wake him up."

"Tom! The police are here! They want to speak to you!"

"Tell em to fuck off will you!" Twisting round to see whether they had heard him, I flushed. From their expressions, they evidently had.

"Don't be stupid." This time I ascended several of the steps. "Get up!"

"I can't," he whined.

"You'll have to. *Now!*" I bolted up the remainder of them until I was bawling at his huddled form from the landing.

Finally he emerged, dragging himself downstairs and towards his would-be captors.

"Tom Clifford," announced the female officer. "We're arresting you on suspicion of burglary. You do not have to say anything but anything you do say might be used in evidence." I knew these words well. The policeman handcuffed him.

"*Burglary!*" I leaned against the wall. "I might have known *he'd* be involved!"

"It's the one at the Spar last night that we want to speak to him about. But there *are* several others. Come on Tom, get your shoes on."

"But I'm not feeling too clever." He looked dreadful!

"Well a nice lie down in the cell should bring you round." The officer turned to me. "Can I ask that you make your way down in about an hour?" He checked his watch as he spoke. "We'll hopefully be ready to interview him by then."

It was a balmy summers evening. Every eye in the neighbourhood was on Tom, as

he was marched out in handcuffs. Watching from the window, I jumped as the van door slammed behind him. The engine roared out of the street and died away, like all my hope. I rang Martin.

"What did I tell you?" It irked me that he sounded almost triumphant. "I knew he was up to something. He's not even been badgering us for money as much over the last few days!"

Half an hour later, Martin arrived home.

"I called into the shop on my way back. It was *definitely* Tom. I've watched the CCTV with my own eyes. You should come back with me and see it for yourself." He rattled the car keys at me. "Just so you're not in any doubt."

"I couldn't." Continuing with my ironing, I slammed the iron down each time, in an effort to dispel my frustration. "What would the owner think of me?"

"He was OK with me. It's not *us* who burgled him!"

"I daren't!" Grabbing one of Tom's t-shirts from the pile, I felt desolate at the Lynx smell that lingered on it.

"I *want* you to see it. There's him and another lad."

In the end I gave in and reluctantly switched off the iron.

Within minutes, I gingerly opened the boarded-up door.

Thankfully the shop had no customers.

"This is Tom's mum," Martin announced, with an air of importance.

"I-I'm sorry," I stammered, unable to look at shop keeper. "I can't believe he's broken into your shop. I'm ashamed of him!"

"It wouldn't happen in our culture. We Sikhs, we make sure our children not bored." The way he surveyed Alex as he spoke conveyed his expectance that he too, would turn out like Tom. "Plenty to do, you see."

Martin spoke again as he gestured up to the security screen. "Can you show her the tape?"

It was so grainy that for a moment I fretted that the Crown Prosecution Service would declare it as not reliable enough evidence, as they had previously. There was no doubting it was him though. Despite the fact that he had attempted to conceal his face in his hood, I could tell from his stature, his movements, his clothes. And I would be more than willing to say so in court too.

"I'll do everything within my power to make sure he's punished for this," I assured the shopkeeper before we left.

At the police station I had to hang around for ages before they interviewed him. It was like waiting to be hung, drawn and quartered.

This time, Tom had requested the services of a solicitor, which took me by surprise. Eventually he arrived, pin-striped and brisk. The desk sergeant indicated to him that I was Tom's mother and perhaps I should be included in their pre-interview discussion.

"I don't think that's a good idea," I decided, remaining firmly in my seat. "You're paid to defend Tom. I'm not on his side whatsoever. I'm only here because I *have* to be."

"Right, OK then." The solicitor seemed a bit taken aback.

As it was, he did not make any difference to the interview and hardly uttered a word.

"Where were you this morning at 1:07 am?" The officer referred to some notes before him.

"In bed," Tom nodded in affirmation.

"Can you verify this?" he continued. "For the benefit of the tape, I'm directing this question to Tom's mother.

"N-no. It was after 4 o 'clock in the morning when he returned home." Tom glowered at me.

A duplicate tape showing Tom entering the shop and stuffing his jacket full of beers and spirits was played on the overhead portable.

"Is this you?" The officer asked him, widening his eyes.

Tom nodded miserably, his whole stature portraying his defeat.

I would now like to move onto your whereabouts on the evenings of the 5th July at around 2am, the 29th June at around midnight and the 27th June at around 1.30 in the morning?" The stuffy room quietened apart from the continual whirring of the tape. I spent a few moments trying to calculate which days of the week they were referring to. I was able to provide an alibi for two of the dates.

"As far as I know he was in bed. But the thing is with Tom, that even after the house is locked up for the night, he will climb out of windows if he wants to get back out." Tom's expression was thunderous. "So I can't provide a *cast iron* alibi."

"Fair enough." The policeman scribbled something down. "We'll see how the CPS respond to that."

In the end he was charged with one count of burglary. His court appearance was less than a week away, on the same day as he had been summoned for non-attendance at appointments with his youth offending worker, one in the morning and one in the afternoon. With a sinking heart, I acknowledged that I was in for a long, drawn-out day.

I went equipped with a bag full of reading matter, sandwiches and a flask of coffee! But I was to be mortified with humiliation as we were frisked upon arrival at the court.

"You can't take those in with you," stated the court official flatly, removing my flask and mug from my bag.

"Why ever not." Several onlookers sniggered.

"Because they could be used as weapons, why do you think?" He locked them into a cupboard. *Of course, why didn't I think of that!*

"Do I look like the sort of person that would use a flask as a weapon? No, on second thoughts, don't bother answering that!"

I was kindly permitted to retain my spoon!

"The case is adjourned for pre-sentence reports," declared the magistrate, looking somewhat bored. "You will return three weeks from today. Your mother will attend with you. All rise."

Sighing, I compliantly rose. I was sick of the sight of these places. Never in my life had I been on the wrong side of the law, yet I was being ordered about like a criminal!"

The Subsequent Court Appearance

Grimacing inwardly, I listened to Tom as he was regurgitated his repertoire to the courtroom. Staring straight ahead, I tried to concentrate on the glimmers of sunshine permeating the gloom through the skylight. It was heartening to be reminded of the beautiful day beyond the confines of these walls. I could not wait to get back out there.

"I don't know what I was thinking. I just followed the others." Tom was heaping regret and sincerity into his voice. "I'll never do anything like it again."

"What *do* you want to do with your life Thomas?" From the expression on his face, the magistrate seemed genuinely interested.

"I want to make something of myself." Tom swept his eyes over the entire courtroom as if ensuring everyone was paying attention. "I just want to get my head down at school and get a good job and stay away from all the idiots I know."

"Do you not think that you, yourself, are indeed an idiot?" I stifled a chuckle.

"Yeah, I mean yes, but I'm gonna change." He stood up straight. "You'll never see me in this court again, I promise!"

"Good because if I do, you'll not be leaving through that door, you'll be leaving through that one." He gestured behind us to a door behind the witness box. "Remember," he went on, wagging his finger. "If you return to this court, you might as well bring your toothbrush with you!" *Gosh, two 'warnings' in one!*

This time he was sentenced to twelve hours at an attendance centre, as well as an extension of twelve months to his supervision order. There was, of course, a fine imposed of £115, payable by my good self!

I could Also Have Papered the Walls with These!

Magistrates Court
Division: 135
Case Number: 14099874638

The Court has found Mr Thomas Clifford guilty of the offences shown below under Offences and Penalties and ordered you as his parent or guardian to pay £115.00.

Date   Offences and impositions
15 Jul 2009 1 / Burglary other than dwelling – theft.
    Comp   30.00
    Costs   85.00
Time to pay: £5.00 per week commencing 18 July 2009
    Total   115.00

The Court has made a Collection Order to collect the sum due.

Application for further time to pay can be made to the Court in person or by post stating fully the grounds on which the application is being made. Alternatively you can contact the Fines Officer on the number above and speak to a member of the fines team. Failure to pay as ordered will make you liable for further enforcement. This could include:

    Deductions from your earnings or benefits
    Increasing your fine by 50%
    Clamping, removal and sale of your vehicle
    Registering the account in the Register of Judgments, Orders and Fines (affecting your ability to obtain credit)
    A distress warrant being issued to the Court Bailiffs for the seizure of goods (incurring additional costs)
    Continued default – imprisonment

A Warning to all Youths

Twelve hours in an attendance centre. A deterrent you might think. What is an attendance centre? Allow me to explain.

- It is held within a school building. Well this one was.
- Tom had to attend there on a Saturday morning between 10 am and 12 am.
- On one occasion the supervising officer was unable to gain access to the school building so Tom was sent home and two hours of time were 'quashed!'
- According to Tom, the two hours were passed in a variety of ways.

1. Watching videos
2. Playing pool
3. Playing table tennis
4. Playing darts
5. Playing dominoes and other table top games
6. Having 'circle time' to talk about feelings
7. Completing worksheets

Alex's Parents Evening

"Are you aware that Alex occasionally discusses things going on for him at home?" I felt flustered as Mrs Smith's question sank in. *Oh no! What had he been saying!*

"No. But I guess he's got to vent it somewhere." I tried to meet her eyes. "He puts up with an awful lot from his brother."

"So I gather!" she smiled. "Has there been any improvement on that front, or are things still as hard?"

"I'm afraid not. We do our best to shield Alex from it but it's not always possible."

"He *does* appear to take it all in his stride." Her smile broadened. "He's quite remarkable!"

"I know. He's a little star." I gestured towards the seat where I knew he sat in class. "He knows about things, and has heard words that no seven-year-old should ever be exposed to."

"Well you'll be pleased to know that his brother's influence is not affecting him at school."

"It's not at home either. I think it's having the opposite effect actually. Alex vows he'll never be *anything* like Tom!"

"We're pleased with him here. He's hardworking, contributes eagerly to discussions and he's doing well."

"That's fantastic!" Her praise of him made me feel warm inside.

"You should be proud of him. He's helpful, polite; if I had a class full of Alexs, I would be a very happy teacher!"

"What about friends? Is everything OK there?"

"Oh yes. There's no one he doesn't get along with. There's one or two boys he spends more time with than others, but no, you've nothing at all to worry about!"

Tears sprang to my eyes. "You don't know how brilliant it is to come here and hear you praising one of my children. It's such a different story to the parents' evenings I have experienced with my eldest!"

"I can imagine!" She put her hand on my arm. "It's been an absolute pleasure to give you such a positive report."

Arrest Number 8

Hello this is a message for Tom's Mum. It's his youth offending worker. Just returning your call. Apparently you wanted to check Tom turned up for his appointment. I can confirm he has – he left the office about twenty minutes ago. If you can ensure he keeps attending and remains out of trouble then that should keep him out of court. Call me back if you need to talk further, bye for now.

About thirty minutes later my phone sprang back into life.
"Is that Tom's mum?" It was a voice I did not recognise.
"It is." He could *not* have been arrested: he had only just left his appointment.
"This is PC Lawrence. I'm just ringing to let you know we picked Tom up about quarter of an hour ago."
"Picked him up! Are you sure? He's been at a youth offending appointment."
"Well it doesn't seem to have done him much good." There was a sneer within his voice. "We got a call from Boots. He was caught trying to nick a pair of designer sunglasses."
"Oh, I don't believe it."
"We'll need you to come down to the station. Is that OK?"
"Erm yes," Then I remembered. "I mean no, my car's in the garage having a new clutch done."
"Is there anyone who can bring you down?"
"No, not really." For a moment, I felt triumphant, believing I may be able to get out of attending his interview whilst maintaining a clear conscience in doing so.
"What about another relative? Someone who could act as his appropriate adult, instead of you?"
"There's no one." Then I thought back to the first interview he had undergone, after the burglary. "Can't you get someone from the youth offending team to do it? They've done it before."
"It would be simpler and quicker if you attended. What time are you likely to get your car back?"

"Tomorrow."

"Oh. Right. Hang on a minute." There was a bit of scuffling and scratching for a moment as he conferred with someone. "OK, we can't let him out till we've interviewed* and charged him. For that we need *you* here. We'll have to send a car out to collect you."

Gulping, I glanced out of my window. "A police car? But my neighbours ....!"

"I'm sorry." He did not sound it. "It might make the difference between us letting him go today or having to keep him overnight in the cells. The car'll be with you in about half an hour."

Alex and Martin thought it was hilarious. As the *marked* car drew up outside my house, I pelted out to it, in my hopeless quest to avoid the neighbourhood glare. Of course most of the neighbours were tending to their lawns, cars or whatever and my mode of transport was witnessed by all. I resisted the urge to give a queen-style wave as I journeyed out of the street.

The policeman who collected me barely uttered a word as he drove. His driving was appalling. Too fast and too close to the left. On arrival, he rammed the car up the kerb outside the police station, narrowly avoiding a lamppost.

"Er thanks," I offered, climbing out quickly. "Do you know you're on double yellows?"

"It doesn't matter," he grunted dismissively. "We're allowed."

---

*Bog standard interview, bog standard questions: *Were the sunglasses yours to take Tom? Were you intending to pay the shop back Tom? Did anyone give you permission to take them?* We spent all evening there until he was eventually charged and bailed.

A week later, he pleaded guilty in court and received a 'severe' reprimand, a lifetime ban from Boots stores, countrywide, and I, of course, got court costs.

Out of Control

Tom shot towards the stairs. There was something frantic in his eyes as he secreted something up his sleeve.

"What've you got there?" I dropped the laundry basket down.

"Nowt." Unusually, guilt was etched all over his face.

"Show me." He tried to bolt off in the direction of the landing so I raced after him.

"Do one will you," he shouted as I grabbed his sleeve.

"I want to know what you're got."

"Fuck off! Gerroff me!" He tried to shake his arm from my grasp.

Letting go, I re-captured him on another part of his arm. There was a soft bulge and a rustle of polythene.

"Get the fuck off me!" He tried to shove me away with his foot.

"You've got drugs haven't you?"

He had lowered himself to the landing floor and was snarling in rage. Both our hands were fastened around the bag of drugs. Neither of us were willing to let go. Whatever he had, it felt like a sizeable amount.

"Fuck off, fucking whore, fucking get off me!"

Fuelled with anger and determination, I won the battle. I emerged victorious and held the large bag of cannabis aloft. Using my rather limited drugs knowledge, mainly gleaned from the internet, I would guess he had about sixty quid's worth.

"Not in my house!" Muttering the words through clenched teeth, in a robot-like fashion, I lurched towards the toilet.

"Mum, no, please!" There was desperation in his voice.

In hindsight, I should have phoned the police and let them deal with it, but I gave myself no opportunity for logical thinking. In one fail swoop I had despatched the offending bag and flushed it away.

"You stupid slag! Fucking slut!"

His venom echoed in my ears as I began to descend the stairs.

I had been hell-bent in uncovering what Tom was concealing; I had been oblivious to poor Alex observing the 'action' from the foot of the stairs. He looked petrified! Before I had reached the bottom to console him, Tom aimed a glass after me. It skimmed the top of my head and narrowly missed Alex.

Seconds after the smash, Martin burst through the door.

"What the hell's going on?" His eyes lurched from me to Tom to the floor. "I could hear all the carrying on from the bloody street!"

"He had drugs," I gasped. "I flushed them down the toilet. So he chucked the glass." I pointed at the floor. "It nearly hit Alex." Barely able to breathe, I fought to get the words out.

"You've two minutes to clear up this glass!" Martin barged past us into the living room. "Before I launch you out of this house; once and for all!"

Amazingly, Tom obeyed this instruction before retreating to his bedroom, presumably to seethe in solitude.

Through the night, I normally keep a glass of water on my bedside table. Mercifully, on this particular night I proceeded to take a sip *before* switching the lamp off.

"Have you put ice in my water?" There was a 'rattle' within my drink.

Closer inspection revealed my glass to be swimming with shards of broken glass.

"Do you know what damage you'd have done if you'd taken a big swig in the night? Not to mention if you'd swallowed any." Martin looked livid.

"Why did he put it here?" I gawped into the glass. "Why didn't he just throw it in the bin?"

"Why do you think?" Snatching the glass from me, he peered into it. "He wants to injure you. Get his own back for flushing his precious drugs away."

"Don't be daft." I scrunched my face in protest. "I know he's angry but he wouldn't hurt me."

"Wake up Sarah. He's just tried to."

A Different GP

"Can prescribe me something?" On the brink of tears, I slumped before the new gp. "I can't cope anymore. I'm not sleeping and feel exhausted."

"Pills are all very well Sarah but they only mask the symptoms. They don't address the problem. Can you tell me a bit about what's going on for you?"

"I feel so low and out of control." I stared down at my hands. "It's crossed my mind to swallow some tablets, fall asleep and never have to face it all again."

The concern was blatant in her expression. "Is it problems at home? Or is it work?"

"It's mainly my teenage son." I lifted my eyes to meet hers. "The whole thing's making me ill. I can't even face working at the moment." Tears leaked down my cheeks. "I'm a prisoner in my own home."

"Go on." Ripping a tissue from a box beside her, she offered it to me.

"I've had a million problems with him, right through his childhood," I tried to steady my voice through my tears. "But for the last three years, it's been abuse on a daily basis. He's heavily into cannabis and even smokes it in the house sometimes." I dabbed at my eyes. "Then he issues threats if I don't give into his demands for money."

"What sort of things does he threaten you with?"

"Sometimes to keep following me wherever I go." Pausing, I blew my nose. "At others it's worse, like threats to slap me, usually when my husband isn't around, or he'll threaten to smash up the house or my car. He steals from us too. Nothing can be left lying around. And I'm in and out of court and police stations. I lost count of how many times he's been in trouble over the last couple of years."

"You have another child too," she glanced down at her notes. How's all this affecting him?"

"To be honest, Alex copes pretty well and just tries to stay out of Tom's way as he gets bullied otherwise."

"Is it physical bullying."

"Not usually. I'm mostly pretty vigilant. It's more name calling, a bit of shoving perhaps if I don't get there in time."

"How would you feel if I were to make a referral to Social Serv...."

"That's all been tried before," I interrupted quickly. "They apparently only deal with abused children, not kids that are out of control."

"To be fair." She whisked a pen from her desk. "They've a duty to protect your youngest son from your eldest. From what you've told me, he must be witnessing far more than he should."

Miserably, I hung my head. "I feel so guilty. Luckily he never copies the swearing or anything. But what could Social Services do?"

"They could offer respite with Tom." She tapped the pen thoughtfully against her chin. "That would be a start."

"And what about giving me tablets?"

"I'd prefer you to talk to a counsellor before we embark along that route." Rummaging around on her desk, she produced a card which she slid across to me. "Use the opportunity to offload it all. I promise that will be more beneficial than any medication I could offer you."

Professional Number 16 The Counsellor

Spilling my problems felt self-indulgent.

The first appointment was spent giving the counsellor background information about my circumstances. "Tom's taking away our home; our dream. None of the neighbours even speak to us." I rested my elbows on the arms of the easy chair. "I'm too ashamed to even hang out my washing. I've coped and coped but it's all making me ill now."

"Which is why you're here." Reaching over, she patted my hand. "We're going to get you through this."

"I just can't relax anymore." I rubbed at my forehead. "There's never any way of knowing what's coming next. I think he's sensing how stressed out I am and is bullying me even more. I've no fight left."

Unlike previous conversations with other professionals, I was able to consider the effect Tom's behaviour was having upon *me*. The counsellor did not seem to be blaming me and the more I disclosed, the more I felt I could trust her.

"As a child, I was neglected, abused and finally rejected completely." My voice wobbled as I scanned her face for an adverse reaction. "But history is not being repeated which is what the child psychiatrists are implying. The negativity I feel towards Tom overwhelms me with guilt. It's reaching a point where I can hardly bear being in the same room as him."

By my third and fourth appointments, I was definitely making progress.

"The care and concern you have for your son is obvious," she stated quietly. "Rather than it being a case of history repeating itself; I think it's actually a cruel irony that you've been subjected to both a mother *and* a son that have treated you so badly."

My eyes burned with tears which I frantically attempted to blink away. "History has kind of repeated itself. But not in the way the child psychologists have suggested."

"What do you mean?" She leaned forwards in her chair.

For several moments, I grappled for the right words. "I was *forced* to be excluded from my family as a child and *had* to stay in my room and eat my meals alone. Tom excludes *himself*."

"Go on." Straightening up, she appeared to be listening intently to my comments.

"When I was young, my mum would only allow me in the house when my dad was at home. No matter how cold or wet it was, I was locked out. So now, when I lay awake, listening to the wind or rain, fretting about where Tom might be, it just makes it harder because I was driven out in weather like that."

She nodded. "I can see how that would make it all the more poignant for you."

"I only want the best for him." I clasped my hands together. "But I'm terrified that one day I'm going to get a call or a visit, telling me he's dead or something. Sometimes I wish the courts would just lock him up. At least I'd know he was safe then."

"Does he ever open up to you?" As she posed the question, she held her arms apart. "Given you *any* insight into what's going on for him or perhaps where he's going at night?"

"He barely acknowledges me these days. But he's been speaking to a man at the Child and Adolescent Mental Health Service; well, when I can drag him there anyway." My eyes inadvertently flickered to the ceiling. "Usually, he kicks up a stink about going."

"Are you part of that process?" She wrote something down.

"No, I was to begin with but it wasn't working out. I was being blamed for the lot. Now, he's supposed to go on his own. I drive him and wait in the car, but every bribery tactic is needed to get him in the car in the first place!" In spite of the angst the counselling session was making me face, I smiled.

"Why do you think they were blaming you?" Awaiting my reply, she tilted her head to the side.

"They took the easiest option, I think. Finding any answers within Tom was always going to be difficult. It was probably far less hassle to point the finger at the mum who'd had a rough childhood herself, *and* given birth when still quite young." My screwed up face must have portrayed my disgruntlement. "To be honest, I've been disgusted with how they've talked down to me and how easily they've formed opinions without even involving any more of Tom's family, like his dad or step parents."

"If he *was* to open up, and you had the chance to make him listen, what do you think you'd say to him?"

For several moments I pondered. There were loads of things I wished he would listen to. "I guess the biggest one is *please don't throw your life away.*" I looked at the counsellor. "He could have such a successful life if he wanted it. He's bright, intelligent, not to mention a lovely looking lad and really, I'd support him to the end of time if he'd give me half a chance."

"And what would you hope to say to him in the future?" Her hand gestures supported her as she spoke. "Let's say in about ten years from now."

"I want to be proud of him; I never have been proud. That's terrible isn't it?" I wrung my hands as I spoke. "I'd love to be able to say. *I'm proud of the way you've turned your life around.*"

"You've proven there, that it's not all negativity." She smiled again.

I shook my head. "But it's only one way traffic. He doesn't care at all about me, or his stepdad, or even his little brother." My voice trailed off. "All he wants me for is whatever he can gain. I honestly can't foresee him *ever* turning his life round or there being an end to any of it. There's a real danger of him dragging me, well all of us, down with him if we allow it."

"You've mentioned feeling *dragged down* or being frightened of being *dragged down* several times." Her hand crumpled into a fist, which she pulled down to rest beside her knees. "What do you mean by it? What is it that you're scared of?"

"The main thing is dissolving into depression. It's bad enough now; but I can't let myself get any worse." My voice shook. What I needed was a good bawl but I wouldn't, or couldn't let go.

"You're stronger than you think," affirmed the counsellor. "Surely you've already proved that to yourself."

"If I get much lower, I'm worried I won't be capable of being a proper mum to Alex. I torment myself about losing my home; or about never being able to return to work. At the moment, my confidence has vanished and there's no way I can even face my neighbours." My gaze flicked to the clock. The appointment was coming to an end. "Who knows what they're all whispering about me."

"But you're not just Tom's mum. You've got to keep hold of that. You're Sarah too."

The GP (again)

"I wanted to see you straightaway," she stated, pointing to a chair. "Have a seat."

Expectantly, I waited for her to continue as I sank down and rested my bag in my lap. "Is it about the referral?"

"Yes." She took a long breath. "I've had a bit of a shock, to be honest."

"Why?" I felt momentarily hopeful. "Are they going to provide some help?"

"No." Her face bore an expression of discomfort. "Quite the opposite in fact. As I promised, I rang them and outlined your predicament to a 'duty' social worker. Firstly she told me that they wouldn't be able to pursue the referral."

"Did she say why?" Listening, I fiddled with the strap on my bag.

"Apparently because Tom is approaching sixteen." She paused. "I explained about your family being at breaking point and the fact you're desperate for respite." She lowered her eyes. "The woman I spoke to was very unhelpful. Eventually, realising I was getting nowhere, I asked to be transferred to someone more senior."

"And?"

"It was the response you'd warned me about. They don't do *anything* to alleviate situations borne out of behaviour issues; they exist solely to prevent child abuse and neglect."

"I've been told that every time."

"But I wasn't happy," she persisted. "I made it clear to this more *senior* person that little Alex should be considered with regard to being bullied *and* his older brother's influence. After a while the woman became annoyed and told me if I wanted to push it, they would just come and remove the youngest one."

"What! She said that! She'd take Alex away!" My heart was pumping madly and I felt dizzy. "They won't! They can't! What are they on about?"

"I was shocked too." She fiddled with paper clips on her desk. "When I asked her to clarify what she meant, she repeated that if I wanted to force them down the child protection route, they would remove Alex, not Tom."

"Did you give them any details about us?"

She shook her head. "Just my name and practice details initially but no, nothing about you, Tom or Alex."

"Can this be left alone?" I heaved a sigh of relief. "I'm scared to death they'll pursue it."

"Don't worry. If they were to come back to me, I'd say the situation's been resolved and we don't require their *help*!"

"Can you promise that nothing more will come of this? You've got me really worried, you know!"

I had been having enough difficulty with sleeplessness and was to manage even less over subsequent nights! The constant dread that lurked within me could not be quelled. *What if they tried to take Alex from me?*

On His Own Doorstep 2

I had not been in bed long. But thanks to two glasses of wine, I was soon dozing off! My body suddenly lurched awake to the intrusion of the doorbell.

On autopilot, I wrapped a cardigan around my bare shoulders and trudged through the darkness to respond. I glanced at the glow of the digital clock. 11:37. *Blimey, he was home before midnight!* That's if it was him, not the police, or a 'hoodie.'

Tom hurtled past me without a word and darted into the living room. As I began to close the door behind him, I heard a peculiar popping noise, coupled with an inaudible angry voice. Tom was peering around the living room curtain.

"What're you doing?"

"Nowt."

Hearing footsteps on the stairs, I realised Tom had woken Martin too. "Can't you hear what's going on out there?" he stormed as he reached the bottom. "It's his bloody mates."

"They're no mates of mine. Not any more."

There was another similar but louder popping noise, then another, then another. Accompanying them was the sound of shattering glass. Flinging the door back open, I was astonished to witness two of Tom's friends beating the hell out of the windows of the house opposite us, with what looked like broom handles.

"Stop it, you idiots!" I screeched, belting towards them in my pyjamas. Somebody had bought this house. Even the 'sold' sign had been uprooted. The thugs had battered three out of four of the double glazed units. One of them brandished his broom handle towards me whilst the other commenced work on the fourth window.

With defiance, I stared into his glassy eyes. Something, other than rage was powering him. "You don't scare me, you know. You're just a little lad. Won't your mum be wondering where you are."

"Get Tom out here!" he demanded.

"Why?"

"Just get him out here!" He was frothing at the mouth. The ghostly faces of our next door neighbours were visible, observing the 'action' from an upstairs window.

There was only me who'd had the gumption (some might say stupidity!) to prevent these hooligans before they wrecked more houses or cars.

"Put the stick down!" Martin strode calmly, but purposefully towards the one still engaged in demolishing the fourth window. "You're both off your heads. You're going to be in some right shit if you don't stop it!"

"I want Tom. Get him out here now!" he insisted through gritted teeth, pausing his frenetic activity for a moment.

"He's a pussy!" stated the other, swaying around as he spoke.

"What do you mean by that?" I was itching to learn what role Tom had played in exacerbating this situation.

"Keep em talking," Martin hissed into my ear. "I've rung the police."

By now they had accomplished their acts of vandalism. One of them sloped down to the ground, apparently exhausted with his efforts. For a few moments, we all gawped at each other, as if wary of the next move.

Then I remembered. *'The security guard!'* Without uttering a word to anyone, I tore off; my sprint slightly impeded in slippers, towards the apartment in which he was usually 'holed up.' Again and again I rang the doorbell. A dim light flickered above. No answer. I began hammering on the door.

"Call yourself a security guard!" I bellowed up at the window. "What a joke!"

At that moment it was flung open. "What you on about? I'm only on duty till midnight. It's well past that!"

"So you just sit back whilst idiots smash in one of the houses! You're a disgrace! You should be sacked!"

"I didn't hear owt!"

"Course you didn't! Well you'd better shift your lazy arse out here and help us keep hold of them till the police get here?"

"I'll be down in a minute." His head disappeared and the window slammed.

It was more like five minutes before he turned out to help. There was still no sign of the police that Martin had dialled 999 for. Both teenagers seemed subdued. One remained slumped on the ground and the other was propped against the garden fence. Clearly they were merely idiotic boys who were out of their depth. Their antics must have been heard streets away; the night was so quiet, even the smallest sound, such as a cat scuttling through its flap was audible.

There was no sign of Tom. Although he had taken no active part in the smashing of these windows, I realised he was must be at least partially responsible for the aggravation of these boys to. The way they had pursued him up our street suggested so anyway.

"What have you taken?" I The 'slumped lad's' face had turned visibly paler in the glare of the streetlamp.

"A bit of this." He struggled to focus on me. "A bit of that. Dunno. Can't remember."

"Why've you done this?" Martin gestured towards the smashed double glazed units. The *security guard* stood over him, in case he made a bolt for it. But to be honest, I doubt he would have had the energy.

"My head went." His head was actually lolling to one side. "Can't take the pressure any more."

Twenty minutes after Martin had made the call, the police finally appeared in a riot van.

"Fucking bitch! You never said you'd rung the filth!" Martin battled to maintain a grasp on him as the van screeched up beside us. The security guard caught hold of the other as he attempted to rise to his feet. Three police men leapt out of the van and sprinted towards us.

"About bloody time too," I jeered, clapping my hands. "It's fortunate that we've managed to do your job for you and keep hold of them."

Two officers had one of the lads pinned to the floor. Squealing like a mouse fastened in a trap, he was being crushed by the force of their weight. Clearly, he had got a burst of energy from somewhere! As they weighed upon him, one of them plucked an aerosol from his pocket. I realised it was CS gas.

"No!" pleaded a voice from somewhere within me. "Don't spray him with that!" His finger poised over the trigger of the can. "Surely three of you can get handcuffs on two drugged up lads, without having to resort to that."

The aerosol was replaced in his pocket. As the handcuffs were clicked on, all fight seemed to drain from him, like a washed-up fish, finally admitting it is beached.

In contrast, the other lad was going quietly.

"Can I have a drink of water?" he pleaded, seemingly directing the question towards me. "I feel like crap."

"Can you hell." The security guard sneered in response to this request as he yanked him towards the van by the hood. "You're off with them!"

"Just a minute. I'll get him one." Crossing the road to our house, I found Tom still cowered behind the curtain.

"You've got some explaining to do in a minute!" I informed him, striding towards the kitchen.

The two lads were taken off and an officer came inside to take a statement.

Tom feigned complete ignorance to the situation and claimed not to even know the lads, even though I knew for a fact that they had called for him on several occasions.

"Can I ask," the officer turned to me as I showed him out, "Why on earth did you prevent us from gassing that thug......and give the other one a drink?"

"They didn't seem in control of any of their actions, not from what I saw. I've got two lads myself, as you know. And that's what *they* are." I glanced across the road at the damage they had caused. "Under all that crap, they're still someone's lads."

Facts About Me

Alex

1. I am 8.
2. My favourite place to swim is Waterworld.
3. I like to spend time on my play station.
4. I am a member of Club Penguin.
5. I enjoy going to cubs.
6. I have got a cute dog.
7. I have got the worst brother in the world.

Why My Brother is the Worst Brother in the World

1. He has stolen so many things from me.
2. Yesterday, he slammed the door on my head.
3. He is an idiot.
4. I don't like him any where near my dog.
5. Because of him, we only have half a happy family.
6. Even my teachers have to know about him.
7. He hurts me and squishes me.
8. I don't like him.
9. He says things that are unkind.
10. He watches weird things on TV.
11. He won't let anyone else watch TV.
12. He is always swearing.
13. He is awful to my mum.
14. Once, he made me actually swear back at him.

Grappling for Survival

"What's wrong with your nose?" Martin screwed his in disgust. "I can't believe you can't smell it!"

I wrenched laundry from the washing machine. "I can."

"So what're we going to do about it?" Standing with his hands on his hips, he surveyed me as though I should have a solution.

Exasperated, I abandoned the washing basket, stormed upstairs and began thumping at the bathroom door.

"Get rid of that now! Or I'm ringing the police!"

"Course you are!"

I am not sure what was worse; the potent hum of cannabis, or the stench drifting from his bedroom. His bedroom door was wide open, expulsing aromas of strongly perfumed deodorant, stale socks, sour milk, old food and who knows what else! The room looked like a cesspit. Only the day before, Tom had moaned that there were no glasses in the kitchen cupboard. I counted nine in his bedroom now. All partially filled with rotten milk or spat in. Cigarette ends floated in three of them. The floor was strewn with rubbish and dirty laundry. His bin overflowed with half-eaten food. Even his bed linen bore the brunt of meals taken upon it and cigarette burns. It had been two weeks since I had last attempted to restore any order in there.

"Are you mad?" had been Martin's question, watching me gag as I scrubbed an undistinguishable substance off his windowsill. "He's going on for seventeen. If he wants to live like a pig, then let him."

So for two weeks I had resisted the urge to go in there altogether, even to remove pots, rubbish and clothes. Deep down I knew Martin was right. I clicked the door shut and returned to the kitchen, furious.

"Sarah, calm down!" Martin poured me a glass of wine.

"How can I? Have you seen the state of his room?" I threw my hands in the air. "Or smelt the stink up there? I've got an asthmatic son asleep in the next room! It's not as if Tom can even be reasoned with. He just does what he wants. I want him out of here! I do! I've had enough!"

"What do you think you're playing at Tom?" Martin asked when he appeared in the kitchen a short time later.

"Smoking a bit a weed in the bath." He flung the microwave door open to inspect his evening meal.

"*My* bath, *my* house!" I rammed a pan into the dishwasher. Martin shot me a look.

"If I smell it in my house again, it won't be *me* banging on the door." I banged the dishwasher shut. "It'll be the police."

"It's a bit of fucking weed!" He swung the microwave door till it slammed closed.

"It's a class b drug!" I screeched, wrestling with the urge to throttle him.

"You chat shit Mum." He programmed the microwave. "You don't know what you're on about. They'd have to find it on me first."

"Just get your tea and quit while you're ahead Tom." Martin strode from the kitchen.

As his tea microwaved, Tom started opening and closing doors to cupboards and the fridge.

"What're you looking for now?" I demanded.

"Summat to eat."

"You've got a pork chop meal reheating in there." I pointed towards the microwave. "You don't know how lucky you are, having a meal waiting for you every night. It was cooked over four hours ago. I must be a right mug!"

Smirking, he stuffed two bags of crisps into one pocket of his 'trackies' and a handful of biscuits into the other. He added three yoghurts, an ice lolly, two bananas and a breakfast bar to his tray. I then observed as he filled a pint glass till it was brimming with milk, greedily necked it, before refilling it.

I jumped slightly as the microwave pinged. The pork chop aroma had thankfully overcome the chemical cannabis smell. Adding the steaming plate to his laden tray, he headed towards the stairs.

"Are you sure you've got enough to eat Tom?" I stared at the tray in disbelief. "I wouldn't want you to feel hungry or anything."

"Leave it Sarah," Martin advised, shaking his newspaper open. "It's the cannabis making him think he needs all that. You should be used to it by now."

Another plate and glass to add to his collection. I fumed, inwardly, worrying that the consumption of so much food and milk at one sitting might make him sick in the night.

My heart sank the next morning because it was only 7.20 when I heard him shuffling around. I preferred for him to sleep in. Quickly, I got dressed, knowing he would be downstairs, bullying Alex if left unattended. However I wasn't fast enough! Hearing him bawling and swearing, I hurtled down the stairs. The dog bolted past me as though she were a squirrel outrunning a predator! As she cowered behind my bed, Alex tore after her, eager to explain.

"Tom was playing with her," he panted. "She was giddy and she jumped up at him. I think she hurt his ear with her paw. But it was an accident!"

"So he screamed at her like that! Tom!" I leant over the banister, "please stay away from the dog in future!"

"She's a little bitch!" He appeared at the foot of the stairs. She's lucky I didn't boot her."

"You hurt my dog and I'll…….." gasped Alex.

"You'll what, you little div?" Tom took a couple of steps up the stairs but then paused. "Shut your ugly little trap!"

"How can you talk to him like that?" I closed my eyes as if hoping to shut his words out. "He's your little brother!"

"I wish I wasn't." Alex folded his arms. "When I'm older and tougher than him, I'll sort him out then."

At this point, I should probably have offered words of correction but I could see where he was coming from.

The door banged a short time later, indicating Tom's departure from the house. I heaved a sigh of relief then felt guilty for it. This was my way of life. Relief when he went out, a plummeting heart when he reappeared. It was not right and these feelings provoked continual guilt within me. Sagging down next to the patio doors I basked in the sudden peace. This was to be shattered by the abrupt barking of the dog. My cup clattered to the floor as I noticed a youth, about Tom's age, scaling along the high wall which bordered my back garden.

"What do you think you're doing?" I flung the door open.

"Looking for me bike."*

"Did you not think to ring the doorbell and ask rather than trespassing?"

*We had warned Tom that no bikes were to be brought back to our house. There had been three in as many weeks, probably stolen.

Fear of Reprisals

I was living on a knife edge. Each time collective voices were audible outside, it probably yielded a gang of hooded youths. Sometimes Tom was among them, at others it would be his 'friends' congregating outside our door in pursuit of him. If car engines were revving manically, it was usually one of his reckless driver friends.

The rear of the house remained locked and I leapt at the doorbell each time it sounded. Usually a sneering hoodie would lurk behind the door.

This time though, I answered the door to yet another policeman. My gaze dashed past him and scanned the street for onlookers before ushering him in.

"What's he done now?" I switched off the tv.

"We've had a complaint from the proprietor of the local off-licence." The policeman loomed large in my living room doorway. "Apparently Tom has been captured on cctv concealing two large bottles of cider under his jacket."

"Oh for God's sake!"

"The shopkeeper was too afraid to challenge him. Apparently there was a large gang of them outside the shop. So he rang us instead."

"Well I don't know where he is at the moment. I can let you know when he gets back."

"That won't be necessary. The shop keeper doesn't want to press charges."

"Why not?"

"He's afraid of the consequences." He shrugged his shoulders. "Having his windows put through.

that sort of thing."

"That's dreadful. God, I'm so ashamed of him."

"Well that's why I'm here." He ventured further into the room.

"To give you the opportunity to put

things right. If you cover the cost of the cider, no more will be said."

"Are you joking? So he thieves and I reimburse it." I pointed at myself. "But he'd just do it again. It could even become an informal arrangement between me, him and the shopkeeper!" I laughed, hollowly. "No! I'll tell him to go back and pay back the cost of the cider himself, but I certainly won't be covering it!"

"Do you think he'll agree to that?" The policeman surveyed me, wide-eyed.

"Of course not!" I snorted. Which is why the shop keeper should press charges. And you should make sure he and his shop are protected. Let the courts bloody deal with him!"

"Well, we can't force him to press charges. But I'll have another word."

In the end Martin went round to speak to the shop keeper. Tom, of course, had sniggered in our faces when we had ordered him to pay for his theft.

"Don't ask for a penny for the rest of the week" I warned. "I'll be giving the money to the shop instead!"

He didn't seem to care. Instead as soon as my back was turned, he snuck a bottle of wine and several cans of beer from the fridge, as well as two of Martin's new blu-ray DVD's.

Martin was grim-faced when he returned from the shop.

"Do you know how embarrassing that was?" He slammed the door. "You can go next time!"

"I'm sorry." I dropped my hands into my lap.

"*You're* his mother!"

"I couldn't have gone in. I'm too ashamed."

"Well the little shit has been back in the shop today. I don't know how he has the nerve! When they refused to serve him, he spat all over the window!" His voice was ascending with every word. "I've ended up having to clean it off!"

A Losing Battle

"Why're you so tight?" Tom yanked a glass from the cupboard and banged it onto the worktop. "It's only a pair of fucking trainers?"

"You don't deserve them. Get off your backside and find a Saturday job! You want trainers." I slammed the bottle of squash in front of him. "You buy them!"

That evening he returned home wearing muddied socks.

"Where're your trainers?" I enquired, glancing up from my magazine.

"I lost em."

I laughed. "How do you lose a pair of trainers?"

"I got em stuck in mud." He began peeling his socks from his feet.

"Well, you'll have to wear your old ones." Trying to feign an air of indifference, I returned to my
magazine.

"I sold em to my mate ages ago."

"Tough." I was bubbling over with fury, though I fought not to show it! "You think you can chuck a perfectly decent pair of trainers away and I'll buy you new ones!" My blood pressure must have been going through the roof!

"Sarah, you daft sod!" interrupted Martin, slamming the remote control down. "Of course he's not
lost his trainers. They'll be hidden in the garden somewhere."

"They're not," Tom asserted, with a smirk.

"Well, you're gonna be walking around in your socks then, aren't you?" I nodded towards the pair he was clutching.

"Well I won't be going anywhere then." His face reddened as he raised his voice. "Not to school, or to my appointments. I'll be here," his finger pointed towards the floor. "And I'll follow you around the house all day, making your life hell until you sort me them."

"Martin have you heard him!" Shrieking, I jumped out of my chair.

"Get out of here now!" he boomed at Tom. "Either up to your room or out of this house. I've had enough!"

"I'm not going nowhere." Tom threw himself into the chair I had vacated. "Not till you get me the trainers."

I stood my ground for two days. Tom's old trainers never reappeared. Some pristine new ones did though. Tearing the box open, Tom grinned in victory. Unable to believe Martin had caved in to him, it was a further two days before I spoke to either of them. I was furious!

<u>At Risk of Losing Another Home</u>

Dear Mr and Mrs Pearson,

We refer to the anti-social behaviour contract that was signed by yourselves when your son, Thomas first offended last year.

It would seem that despite the cautions that police officers have issued, he continues to behave in a way that contravenes the terms of the behaviour contract.

We would draw your attention to the following behaviours, many of which are affecting the local community and have invited complaint:

- Using foul and offensive language whilst in public.
- Climbing on the property of other people.
- Entering private gardens.
- Graffiti.
- Acting in a drunk and disorderly fashion.
- Urinating against people's fences.

Indeed he has recently been the subject of a complaint where a local resident, upon finding Tom in his garden, was verbally abused and subjected to Tom urinating against his front door after he had returned inside.

You will agree that this form of behaviour in the local community is unacceptable and as such, we have a duty to inform your landlord. As you will no doubt be aware, you are responsible not only for your own conduct, but for that of anybody who resides with you or visits you.

The next step in our proceedings will be to refer your family to the court with a view to obtaining an anti-social behaviour order. <u>This will inevitably result in the loss of your tenancy as you will invariably be in breach of your tenancy agreement.</u>

You may, at this point, wish to take advice from a solicitor or the Citizens Advice Bureau.

Yours sincerely

Anti Social Behaviour Unit

Don't Call Me Mum!

(15 years, 10 months)

The following morning, I dropped Alex at school before embarking on the ten minute drive towards Tom's pupil referral unit.

"Stay there," I ordered as he unclipped the seatbelt to get transfer himself into the front seat after Alex had got out. "I don't want you sat at the side of me. Not after the letter I've had!"

"I don't even know why you're taking me to fucking school." He rammed his fist against the back of the passenger seat. "I'm not going in." He was always at his absolute worst on a morning and had, today, surfaced in the darkest of moods.

"You *are* going in!" I pulled up sharply at a junction and twisted my neck to glare at him. "Do you think I can cope with *you* at home all day?"

"Well you'd better be giving me some money then." Sinking back in his seat, he folded his arms.

"You must be joking." My voice heightened in pitch. "After the letter we've had?"

"*What* letter?"

"Weren't you listening last night? The letter threatening to throw us all out."

"Oh that letter. Nah, I wasn't listening." He looked out of the window. "Just thought you were ranting again."

"Ranting!" I rammed at the button for the car radio to turn it off. "I have every right to. I'll give you ranting!"

"So do I get some money or what?" He leaned forward.

"Tom, do you realise what you're doing to us?" I battled to keep my eyes on the road. "We might all be getting kicked out because of you."

"You're chatting shit again Mum!" He looked impatient. "Course we won't get kicked out!"

"After the way you've been carrying on!" Wrenching the letter from my pocket, I hurled it behind me so it landed on the back seat. "What'll we do if we lose our house! I can't believe you don't care about it!"

"I just want money." He didn't even look at the letter. "I'm not getting outta the car until I've got some!"

"You bloody are!"

"|Make me."

"Tom you're getting no more money from me. You can forget it."

"F**king tight b-i-t-c-h!" As the last word escaped him, he booted the back of my seat as ferociously as he could.

Screeching the car up to side of the road, I lashed back at him, my flailing arm failing to connect with his irritating head. "I'm sick of you talking to me like that!" I began to cry, mainly with unexpressed rage. "I can't take any more of you."

"Stupid cow. Sort yourself out."

"How can you talk to me like that?" I rested my arms, then my head against the steering

wheel. I don't know how you live with yourself."

"Quite easily."

"You'll know about it when you're older and you don't have anyone." I wrenched my head

back up. "You're a nasty piece of work! Don't think I'll take this off you forever." I resumed the journey and drove for the final stretch in silence. Pulling up outside the pupil referral unit, I waited.

"What are you doing?" He did not move. "I'm not getting out. Are you deaf or summat?"

"Get out of this car before I launch you out!" I thumped the steering wheel.

"Give me some fucking money Mum, now!"

"Don't call me mum! Don't you bloody call me mum! You've no right. Not with the way you treat me!"

In the end I hurled four pound coins through the window of the passenger seat. He darted from the car to gather them up, allowing me the opportunity to speed away without having to hear what he shouted after me. Hatred bubbled up and escaped through my eyes as tears. I hated him but hated myself more for hating him. *What sort of a mother was I?*

In a trance, I drove on. There was no way I could go on living with him. Bit by bit, I was being destroyed. At that moment, I decided to *force* the authorities to help. Yes. I would inform them that he could not return home that evening. That I had reached breaking point. It would be better for us all this way. Especially him. If you flick back to the opening chapter of this book, part of the phone call I made is included there.

Letter to the MP

29 October 2009

Dear Mr Gregory,

Your secretary advised me to provide information about my circumstances prior to our meeting.

I live on the edge of your ward and I rent my house through a housing association. My problem is anti-social behaviour perpetrated by youths in the area, of which my 15-year-old son is one of the ringleaders.

18 months ago, at our previous address, my son began to offend. Firstly, he burgled our next door neighbour. He was arrested, but was about to be released due to lack of forensic evidence. The police were struggling to charge him, so they asked me to speak to him.

I persuaded him to 'do the right thing' and own up. Because of this admission, he was brought to court. However, the court ordered me to pay compensation of £600 to our neighbours and Tom was barely punished.

He then went on to cause over £500 of criminal damage. This was in addition to all the other anti-social behaviour he was displaying in and around the home. This swiftly resulted in a written contract having to be drawn up with the anti-social behaviour team.

Our landlord also asked us to leave the property.

We moved to our new home over a year ago, a move that I, my husband and my youngest son, who is 7, were delighted with. However, Tom has quickly acquainted himself with the local delinquents, and we have just been issued with a written warning regarding his anti-social behaviour which has included being drunk, causing trouble around people's homes, burglary of a shop, shoplifting and urinating against people's doors. We have been told that any further behaviour of this kind will result in us losing our tenancy.

We will be deemed to have made ourselves intentionally homeless as we have failed to control our son, therefore will be unable to secure future social housing.

Since this written warning, Tom has continued to shoplift, drink excessively and has been brought back on two occasions by police. At the weekend, we discovered that a further complaint will now be made to the anti social behaviour team. The police state that Tom is not a just follower within this gang of yobs; he is one of the main perpetrators.

In the last 18 months, I as his mother, have attended the police station with him to act as his appropriate adult on about 9 separate occasions so far and have been to court on about 15 occasions. The court have given him supervision orders and tagging orders, both of which he has breached time and time again, leading him back to court and forcing me to have to pay the costs. I feel the court have not punished him at all for his crimes.

The rest of us, as a family, are peaceful, law abiding people, who have struggled with Tom since infanthood. He was hyperactive and destructive then. School have also battled with him and by high school he was causing vandalism, truanting, bullying, fire setting and smoking cannabis in school. He has no respect for authority and will be verbally abusive when challenged. He now attends a pupil referral unit, having been excluded from school.

This is also the case at home. He bullies his younger brother and is severely abusive to me. This has several times resulted in him issuing threats or causing damage. He towers over me and intimidates me.

We have tried to ensure he complies with his court orders and have attempted every imaginable way of keeping him in the house at night so he cannot go out causing trouble. If we try to ground him, he just laughs in our faces so I have been giving him £2 for each time he comes in on time, in the hope that a financial arrangement may engage him more. 10pm weekdays and 11pm weekends.

After the house is locked up for the night, Tom frequently uses knives to unscrew the window locks and escape.

In addition, he steals from us. We have to carry valuables around on our persons and keep things such as the lap top and camera locked away. He has sold most of his own possessions and many of ours. A couple of these thefts were reported to the police but we were made to feel like timewasters.

Over the years we have seen various child psychologists and specialists; sought help from the 0-19 team 3 times, the Child and Adolescent Mental Heath Team twice, we feel let down by the courts, although the youth offending team is supportive.

Social Service's help has been repeatedly sought, especially in view of the fact that Tom's conduct, particularly at home, has a detrimental effect on my younger son. My GP tried to obtain help for us with Tom from Social Services recently, but was informed that if she wanted to pursue the case for my younger son, social workers would simply come and remove him!

I feel desperately 'failed by the system' and am worried about the threat of us losing our home. I have employed many approaches, both recently and in the past but our family is now at breaking point. He loiters around outside our house with large gangs of hooded friends and we are obviously finding ourselves ostracised from our neighbours. Attempts to move his friends on are met with threats and taunts.

As the local MP; you will be aware of the problem with anti social behaviour and will be keen to stamp it out. If we were a family condoning his behaviour, I would expect eviction from the community. But we are as powerless as the local shopkeeper who dares not press charges against those who shoplift from him in case his shop windows are smashed in.

Many people have suggested I contact you for assistance. I do not know what to do next and hope you may be able to advise me further.

Many thanks in anticipation of your help and your time, I look forward to meeting with you.

I am not sure what I was hoping to achieve with this letter. But I'd fruitlessly sought help from my GP, Social Services, The 0-19 Team and The Child and Adolescent Mental Health Service. I felt utterly failed by the judicial system, and had eventually been advised by various quarters to try our local member of parliament.

Anti social behaviour was riding high in the media and was rife within our local community. I felt sure the MP would be interested in being instrumental in 'stamping it out' within his ward. After all, there was an election looming.

And what better person to have on board for him, than a parent of one of the troublemakers?

"I hope you don't mind me bringing my little boy along?" Alex smiled at him nervously as we stepped onto the thick carpet, sinking into it. Wax polish and expensive aftershave permeated the air. The MP sat prominently behind his desk, sparkling under a grand chandelier.

"It's always a pleasure to meet my younger constituents." He offered Alex a handshake. "So, how can I be of assistance to you?"

"I left a letter with your secretary last week," I explained as Alex and I sat before him. "Our situation would take so long to explain, that the allocated ten minutes wouldn't be enough time. I thought it would help if you already had background information so were aware of our situation before meeting us."

"Ah yes, the antisocial behaviour problem." Glancing at the timer before him, his brow furrowed. "I'm afraid I haven't had the opportunity to read your letter in depth. How old is your son again?"

"Nearly 16. I've already dragged him to a multitude of specialists and got nowhere." Raising my eyes from the lacquered table, I allowed my eyes to meet his. "You're my last hope."

"Well, I'll do what I can, of course." He clasped his fingers together on the table. "But I'm not sure what I can ...."

"It's not as if we've brought him up like this," I persisted. We've tried everything with him. Now he's a teenager, he's becoming unstoppable. And it's worse now he's hanging about with similar lads. They all want stopping." I was gabbling. It was partly nerves, and partly because of the time constraint. "I'm suffering just as much as every one else in the neighbourhood, if not more!"

"Does he have any sort of criminal record yet?"

"You could say that!" In spite of the desperation I felt, I laughed. "It's all in the letter I wrote you. But the police and the courts have done nothing apart from punish *me*!"

"I'm not sure whether...."

"We're going to lose our home!" I was hardly pausing for breath. "They all hang about outside! The police have informed us he's on their 'hit list' for eviction from the area. I don't know what we'll do if we're made to leave!"

"It doesn't seem fair that an entire law abiding family should lose their home because of just one individual. When is he sixteen?"

"In two months." Glancing at Alex, who was perched quietly beside me, I felt guilty at him being subjected to this conversation, however, there had been no one to look after him.

"Ah, well then," the MP slapped his hand upon the table, like a prized fish. "The answer's staring at us! He can secure independent accommodation when he reaches sixteen."

"It's not as simple as that. Who on earth would offer a tenancy to a sixteen-year-old?"

"Is there any family who'd take him in?"

"Of course not!" I bestowed my most withered look towards him.

At least the man was attempting to *sound* helpful! But he was floundering. The outcome I had been seeking was that he would want to throw his weight behind us; and perhaps have influence with the police and housing office.

"Leave it with me." He rose to shake my hand again. "I'll have a thorough look at your letter, make some enquiries and get back to you, hopefully with answers or at least a bit of advice."

A month passed. I heard nothing. The e-mail I sent via his secretary but did not yield a reply either. Obviously the MP was not unduly concerned about the onslaught of antisocial behaviour in his ward.

Arrest Number 9

It had been an exasperating morning; supply teaching with an impossible class. I escaped with my lunch and book to the tranquillity of the car, rather than encounter a staff room bursting with strangers.

In hindsight, my need for solidarity was probably associated with my poor confidence; a street-full of condemning neighbours and a life-time of being ostracised. These combined elements had served to ensure that my self esteem was now at an all-time low.

Chewing on my sandwich in the silence, I decided to ring Martin to check on things at home.

"You must be telepathic." He answered on the first ring. "I was about to call you. Are you sitting down?"

"I'm in the car." I fiddled with the half-eaten sandwich in my lap. "Just having my lunch. Why, what's up?"

"He's been arrested again. His school have just been on the phone."

"Oh, bloody hell!" I leaned my head backwards against the seat. "What's he done now?"

"School found a top-of-the-range sat nav and Blackberry phone on him."

"A Blackberry phone? What's that?"

"They've only just come out. They're like miniature computers and are worth a fortune! Anyway, school wanted to know what Tom was doing with these things so I told them he must of nicked them. Apparently, they were going to confiscate them and let the police know. He's then tried to do a runner but they've managed to hang onto him till the police got there."

"Here we bloody go again! Another evening of fun and games." Catching sight of my reflection in the rear view mirror, I felt depressed as I acknowledged the shadows beneath my eyes.

"Apparently the stuff has been pinched from a car round the corner from our house. It'd been left in the car. He was probably planning to flog it after school."

"But they've got it back now?" I picked at the corner of my sandwich.

"Yeah but they're gonna be asking him about other car thefts that have gone on around here. They say there's been a few."

Police Search 2

"We need to search your house, I'm afraid. It shouldn't take too long." Extracting two pairs of rubber gloves from her bag, she proceeded to pass a pair of them to her male colleague. "Have you had your house searched before?"

I nodded slowly. "Where do you need to look?" I swiftly made a mental assessment of the state my upstairs rooms had been left in. "Everywhere?"

"Mainly in Tom's bedroom. As she spoke, she scanned her eyes around my living room. "To be honest, I'm satisfied we won't find any stolen goods concealed elsewhere, aren't you?" She turned to her colleague.

"Well, yes," he agreed as he wiggled his fingers into a glove, "but we still need to have a quick look around."

I led them up to Tom's room.

"Gosh, it's tidy," she remarked as she entered his tiny bedroom.

"You wouldn't have thought that a week ago." I lingered in the doorway, observing as she tugged a box from beneath his bed. "It was an absolute hovel! But we'd run out of glasses and cutlery and I'd got to a point where I couldn't bear *not* to clean it in here. It wasn't a pleasant job mind!"

"Do these belong to him?" She held up the electronic wires and mobile phone chargers that nestled amongst Tom's bits and pieces.

"No. This one says *Tom-Tom* on it." I pointed towards the logo. "So does that one. They would only work with a sat nav. This one looks like a mobile phone charger though." I scrutinised it. "Nokia. He's never had a Nokia phone."

"Do you know where he got these from?" She reached out and took them from me.

"Of course not!" I felt insulted that she suspected I could have known and not acted on it.

"It looks like he's been busy." She turned to the man, as he ransacked Tom's sock drawer. "Anything?"

"No." He nodded towards the bundle of chargers she clutched. "It looks like that's the lot."

"So what happens now?" I signed the form consenting for the removal of the wires.

"Well we've got the sat-nav and the phone back. But he'll still be charged with theft. We'll be asking him about these wires as well." She slid them into a large polythene bag. "We'll give you a call to let you know when we're ready to interview. Have you been appropriate adult before?"

"Just a few times," I groaned.

* * *

Flinging open the door, I was startled to see an immaculately dressed, unsmiling woman before me. I had expected the police or someone in a hood!

"I'm here about your son." She attempted to look beyond me. "Is he here?"

"No. He's ...," I stopped. "Who are you anyway?"

"I want a word with him." She stepped towards me. "He's robbed our stuff."

"Do you want to come in a minute?" I held the door open. No way was I conducting this conversation in full view of the street. Her expensive perfume drifted up my nostrils as she breezed in and followed me into our living room. My gaze hurriedly swept over the dusty TV, discarded magazines and spent mugs. *I should've tidied up!*

"Have a seat," I offered, beckoning towards a chair.

"No, you're alright thanks." She turned to face me. "I'll stay where I am if you don't mind."

I could feel myself disintegrating.

"You're lucky that *I'm* here, instead of my husband, to be honest." Her tone was icy.

"Look, I can't tell you how sorry I am about what he's done." I stared at her costly-looking patent shoes which burrowed into the pile of the carpet. "But luckily his school caught him with both items and....."

"The sat-nav *and* the Blackberry?"

"Yes. Luckily they phoned my husband. They've confiscated the things and told the police."

"Well thank God for that," she let out a prolonged breath. "My husband was facing the sack. There was all kinds of confidential stuff on that phone. It's not even his, it's the company's. It shouldn't have even been left it in the car."

I hung my head. "He wasn't expecting a thieving toe-rag to come along though, was he?"

"He forgot to lock the car," she continued. "Apparently your son, as well as a few other lads, are prowling around the estate regularly, trying all the car doors."

"Look," I took a deep, slow breath. "The stuff's safe and he's going to get prosecuted. I'm off up to the station soon whilst they interview him."

"Do you think we'll get our things back if I go up?" Her whole attitude towards me seemed to have softened.

"I've no idea, but I don't see why not."

"My husband will be so relieved. It was difficult stopping him from coming round. He'd have torn your son limb-from-limb. He's fuming so he still might, you know."

"Listen," I spoke slowly as I sought for appropriate words. "You've got every right to be angry but can you try and talk your husband down?" I looked at her directly. "My family have been to hell and back in the last couple of years because of my son. We still have no idea where it might end?"

"I've got a lad myself and he'd never dream of pinching." She looked haughty about it.

"He's into cannabis," I tried to explain as though that justified everything. "We've been fighting a battle we can't win. It's not like we aren't trying. Perhaps if he'd been punished by the courts in the first place, we might not be where we are now."

"I feel sorry for you. You seem like a good mother." Glimpsing round my living room, I could see she was scanning frame after frame adorning the walls and surfaces, of grinning images of both my boys at varying stages of their lives.

"I'll speak to my husband," she promised, starting back towards the door. "We'll arrange to get our things returned and as long as your son never comes anywhere near our home again, that should be an end to it."

"Thanks." I went towards her to show her out. "For being so reasonable."

"I hope things improve for you." She turned back before embarking down the path. "It must be difficult."

"It is," whispering to myself, I softly closed the door after her.

In Court Yet Again

"It's your poor mother I feel sorry for." Scanning the face of the magistrate, I tried to fathom whether he was being genuine or sarcastic. "Do you suppose she enjoys trudging back and forth to this court, shamed by yourself, because you have no control over your conduct and your thieving impulses?"

"No, and I'm sorry for what I've put her through." Tom was giving an Oscar-winning performance as usual. He stood, like a soldier 'at ease.' "I'm never going to pinch again and I'm glad I was caught and they've got their stuff back."

"A commendable speech Thomas. But do you actually mean it? I've met your sort before. Many a time, unfortunately."

"Your honour," announced a man, rising up from the 'prosecution' bench. He waited till he was acknowledged before proceeding. "We would request that this matter be referred for a pre-sentence report." He cleared his throat. "We think it appropriate that all options be considered. There are too many previous convictions for this case to be concluded with a simple reprimand and court costs."

"Hmmmm." The magistrate looked thoughtful as he scratched beneath his wig. "Am I correct thinking that the stolen property was fully recovered and returned to its rightful owner?"

"Yes. But we do have concerns that Tom will offend *again* if this incident is treated more leniently just because the property was recovered."

"Very well." He nodded slowly. "I will adjourn for two weeks. In this time a pre-sentence report that considers 'all options' will be prepared by the youth offending service. I will take their recommendations."

"All rise." The usher rose to his own instruction.

"You could get sent down Tom," I warned darkly. "You'd better prepare yourself." Exiting the gloomy court room, we stepped back into the public waiting area. My eyes strained to catch his expression in the seeping sunlight. It was belting through the glass roof, before bouncing up, down, back and forth in the white marble interior where we now faced each other.

"That'd make you happy, wouldn't it Mum?" His face was etched in a scowl.

"Don't be daft. You straightening yourself out would make me happy."

"Don't lie. I'm not bothered if I get sent down anyway. I've got mates in the young offenders place. It's a piece of piss in there anyway." He grinned then. "Just play pool and that."

"Tom." It was a woman from the youth offending team. One who always regarded Tom through rose-tinted spectacles.

"Alright love," he grinned, as he swaggered back towards her.

"I need a quick word before you go. About the pre-sentence report." She smiled at him. "Follow me."

Obediently, we trailed after her, as though drawn by lengths of string, into the room where Tom had received a 'roasting' after his first ever offence. That seemed so long ago now.

"Have a seat." Across the table, she leaned towards Tom.

"Am I gonna get sent down?"

"We've been told to *consider all options* so yes; it is a possibility, if the magistrate decides to go *against* the recommendations of our report. Though, we will be arguing for you *not* to be given a custodial sentence. I don't think it would have a positive effect on your situation at all." She smiled at me then, evidently expecting gratitude.

"Why?" If I was to be honest, part of me wanted him to receive a custodial sentence. Mainly to shock him into sorting himself out, but also to afford us, as a family, some respite. "Every other punishment has been trialled with him. Nothing works."

"Have you fucking heard *her?*" Tom would not even look at me. "She actually *wants* me to get sent down. Some fucking mother!"

"I don't Tom." I sighed deeply. "I just want *you* to get punished for a change. Instead of me."

"We'll be arguing for further reparation and the opportunity for Tom to consider how his offending behaviour affects others," the woman continued, obviously trying to maintain a balance between us.

"An opportunity for him to talk the talk, you mean." Leaning back in my chair, I emitted a fake chuckle. "While I get a fine and court costs again."

"I know this must all be difficult for you but......"

"You've no idea. I'm sick to death of being dragged to this place again and again. And police stations! And getting punished!" I laughed again. "Do you know, I've never committed a crime in my life!"

* * *

The court did go along with the recommendations of the youth offending team. As I had predicted, I got costs and a fine. Tom got further reparation, an order to attend a victim awareness course and an order to attend weekly sessions with a drugs worker. I was heartened about this final sanction but doubtful as to whether Tom would engage with any help around his drug use.

"You should be thanking your lucky stars you didn't get sent down," I wearily asserted to Tom as we left court. "For a moment, I thought those magistrates were considering it. Especially when they 'retired' for ten minutes."

"So did I. Thank fuck I'm outta there!" He strode happily alongside me.

"Tom," I cringed as we passed two women. Their disgust at his language was obvious. "Will you stop swearing in front of me?"

"Look at my new trainers too," he moaned, ignoring me as he raised a foot from the pavement. "One of em's scuffed! Can you take em back and change em?"

"Don't be ridiculous!" Shaking my head, I chuckled. "You can't take trainers back because they're scuffed! You'd be laughed at!"

"Why would I?" He stamped his foot back down. "I've not had em long!"

"Look, I didn't want you to have them in the first place. And I certainly don't want to discuss them!"

For a few moments, we walked side-by-side in silence.

"So, are you gonna give me any money?"

"I can't believe your cheek." I gave him my most condescending stare instead. "I've just been ordered to pay over a hundred quid and you're hounding me for money!" I laughed through my nose. "No chance! Not a good time to ask!"

"Come on Mum." He nudged me in the arm. "Don't be tight."

"I'm not paying those costs anyway. You are." I pointed at him. "You can have a couple of quid a day until I've got them paid off. Then if you stay out of trouble I'll up it a bit."

"A couple a quid! What the fuck am I supposed to do with that like?"

"I wouldn't knock it Tom. I should be saying that you get nothing at all." I reached into my purse and plucked out two pound coins. "Here, that's all you're getting."

"You can shove them up your arse!" He slapped at the hand offering the money.

"Fine." Dropping them back into my purse, I snapped it shut.

"I need some fucking money Mum and if you don't give me any I'll...." He stopped dead in the path of where I was walking.

"You'll what?" Slipping my purse back into my handbag, I winched it higher up my shoulder.

"I'll smash your fucking car up!" He flailed his arm out in the direction of where I had parked it. "Why are you being a dickhead?"

I swung around and faced him. "I've just spent all morning in court, fined yet again and now you're abusing me." I nudged him out of my way. "Get away from me! Get the bus home! Go on! You've got a bus pass!" I pushed him again. "I can't take any more of you!"

"Like the fuck I will, you stupid bitch!" He grabbed my arm.

I swung my bag at him, "Get away from me!" One or two people were watching us. By now I was too angry and upset to care.

"Money or I'm going nowhere!" He still had hold of my arm.

"If you think you're getting in my car you've got another think coming."

"You won't even have a car. I've told you what I'll do." Marching behind me, he was crimson-faced with anger."

"So you're threatening me, are you?" Marching on, I was so upset, I felt winded. "I've a good mind to report you."

"To the police?" He laughed out loud. "Weirdo! What'll they do."

"Leave me alone Tom." By now I was openly weeping but I wasn't bothered. "I'm warning you."

"Or what?" He tugged at the strap of my bag. "You'll hit me with your handbag again?"

We reached the car. I tried to jump in and lock it but he was too swift and leapt straight into the passenger seat.

"Get out of my car!" Screeching, I pushed at his shoulder. "What the hell did I ever do to deserve a son like you?"

"Get a load of yourself! What a fucking state!"

"You've made me like this!"

"Money Mum, then I'll go." He stretched his hand out towards me.

Grappling in my bag, I fished out a five pound note and thrust it at him.

"Is that it?" For a moment, he stared at it, before snatching it away.

"Get out of the car," I couldn't look at him. I just needed him away from me.

For the entire journey home, I wept and am surprised I didn't turn the car over. Tears of guilty hate leaked from me. I sobbed so hard that by the time I got home I felt ill.

It was several hours before I dragged myself from the sofa. And only because of the necessity to respond to the doorbell. Trudging towards it, I wondered what bad news it yielded this time.

"Is Tom in?" I looked from one boy to the other. They were younger than Tom. Amazingly, they didn't have a hood between them, and I was astonished to notice they were both wearing 'proper' trousers and smart shoes. Not the usual appearance of someone calling for Tom!

"Er...no. He's not here at the moment. Who shall I say called?"

They glanced uncomfortably at each other. Then one spoke up. "He's stolen some money from us."

"Has he indeed?" I leaned against the frame of the doorway. "Do you want to tell me a bit more about it?"

The other boy looked down at his shiny shoes, "We're scared of any repercussions," he stated, flatly.

"If Tom *has* stolen from you." I folded my arms, "*he'll* be the one in trouble. How much has he stolen?"

"Twenty pounds." He fiddled with the zip on his bag as he spoke. "My mum's going to kill me."

"How did he steal it? Did you leave your bag somewhere?"

"Kind of," he glanced at his friend.

"When was it taken?" I straightened up then, hoping they would say it was earlier that day, when Tom could not possibly have been anywhere near them.

"About two hours ago."

"Are you sure it was Tom?" I surveyed them again. They were at least two or three years younger than him. "I mean, how well do you know him?"

"Yeah it was definitely him." The other boy puffed his chest out. "Look we don't want any hassle; just our money to be returned. Can't *you* give it to us?"

"Me? Why should I?" I stepped back inside my hallway. "If you're telling the truth and Tom *has* stolen your money, then you need to inform the police. You've nothing to worry about. The police will deal with him."

"But *you* won't give us it?" He looked at me beseechingly.

"No. But, listen, I'm on your side. If Tom's stolen from you, he should be punished. Go home and let your parents know what's happened. Let them decide what to do. I'm sorry," I flung my arms in the air. "I can't say any more than that for now."

As they scuttled away, I replayed the conversation in my mind. *Menacing young boys for money!* I waited for him to return so I could confront him.

"It was for cannabis," he smirked, tugging a bag of crisps from the cupboard. "They wanted me to get em some."

"But that makes you a.... a *dealer!*" My hand flew to my mouth.

276

"How does it? I didn't even get em any?"

"So you just accepted their money and pocketed it?" I slammed the cupboard door that he had left ajar.

"No, I've spent it," he spoke through a mouthful of crisps.

"Well if they've told their parents, you'll be having a visit from the police soon." I glanced up at the clock.

"As if they'll have told anyone!" he chuckled, extracting a carton of juice from the fridge. "That they wanted to buy weed!"

My eyes travelled to his feet. "What have you done with your trainers?"

He took a large gulp from the carton. "I swapped the scuffed one?"

"How?"

"In the shoe shop." He wiped his mouth. "The one on display was my size, lucky eh?."

I shook my head, incredulously. He had left court, after making all his declarations of 'change,' been vile towards me, fleeced two boys out of twenty pounds and stolen a trainer!

Arrest Number 9

The next arrest involved a police station I had not yet been acquainted with; it was located in the centre of town, fifteen or so miles from our house.

"We've got him in custody," stated a male voice, dispassionately. "We need you to be here as soon as possible please."

"What's he done this time?"

There was a pause and a rustling of pages. "He's stolen a bottle of beer from Sainsbury's to the value of £1.46."

"Pardon?" I gripped the phone, thinking I had misheard. "£1.46."

"That's correct."

"But it'll cost me ten times that in petrol and parking." I shook my head. "You've got him locked up for £1.46?"

He exhaled audibly. "I know. And I agree it does seem ridiculous." His voice held a hint of regret now. "If it was his first offence we would just ask you to cover the cost. But because of his already, extensive criminal record, we've *got* to prosecute him."

"I understand," I sighed.

Possibly because it was within the city centre, the police station was even bleaker than the one he was usually confined at. It reminded me of a bustling cattle market. Angry tirades from occupied cells rattled around the walls. Uniforms swarmed everywhere. A stench of stale alcohol hung in the air, made worse by two drunks I watched being dragged in. They were so inebriated; they had to be supported to stay upright whilst their rights were read to them.

In a bid to pass the time, I studied the 'guest list' of occupied cells. The spaces next to cells 24 and 41 advised *do not use, to be steam cleaned.* Nice.

Before long I was joined on my bench by a man whose son had been *wrongly* incarcerated after a neighbourly row. I was treated to a rendition of his entire life story as well as recount of the whole evening of his evening. Nodding politely, I was aching to tell him to get lost and leave me alone! Eventually, a policewoman took pity on me.

"We'll put you in the interview room for a few minutes until we bring Tom through." She led me into one of the all-too-familiar airless green rooms. "I thought you needed rescuing!"

"You're not kidding!" I smiled at her gratefully. "Thanks!"

An alarm wailed through the station like a wounded animal. The officer, along with an array of identical uniforms hurtled towards one of the cells. It was surreal, like a scene from the TV. Eventually, she reappeared, with a male officer and Tom, sheepishly clad in paper trousers. He bowed his head in shame as he trudged into the interview room.

"I'm sorry Mum." He slumped beside me, his paper trousers rustling with the movement. "I can't believe I've been caught for something so stupid!"

"It's not about being caught!" I blustered, twisting myself to face him. "It's about stealing in the first bloody place!"

"I know."

"Well this shouldn't take long." the policewoman unwrapped the tape and slotted it into the machine. "Right I'm going to start the tape, then read your rights. Do you need them explaining to you?"

"No."

"Off we go then." The recording machine emitted a lengthy beep, signalling the interview had commenced.

I listened peripherally as Tom responded to a series of ludicrous questions.

"Did the beer belong to you?"

"Who did the beer belong to?"

"Did anyone say you could take the beer?"

"What did you do with the beer?"

"Were you intending to go back into the shop and pay for the beer?"

"Whilst you are here," the policewoman glanced down at her notes, "we've also been asked to investigate a complaint about the theft of a firework."

"A firework?" Tom bore an expression that hovered between innocence and puzzlement.

"Yes. A dud firework." She appeared to be stifling a wry smirk. "It was removed from the display of a shop that's opened in the main street where you live. We've got you on cctv trying to light it afterwards."

"Oh for pity's sake!" I wasn't supposed to speak during the interview but the words just came tumbling out.

"Have you anything to say Tom?"

"Yeah, OK. It was me." He slapped the palms of his hands on the table. "But it was me mates too. And it didn't work anyway."

"That's not the point, is it Tom? Stealing is stealing."

He was then replaced in his cell, pending decision by the CPS. I resumed my wait on the metal bench. The man smiled as I retook my position. His son's predicament had developed in the time that had elapsed. *Come on, hurry up!* I prayed silently as his whisky-laced words trickled over me.

"We've highlighted the court date on the sheet," stated the desk sergeant, sliding the sheet towards Tom, now wearing his tracksuit bottoms again.

"He's got to go to court?" I raised my eyes towards the yellow ceiling. "For £1.46 and a dud firework?"

The sergeant then slid another piece of paper towards me, sideward's on.

"For a lad of not even sixteen, his record is astounding." His hand remained on the document as he waited for my reaction.

"I know." I scanned the lengthy list. "And before you start assuming I'm to blame, this is not how he was brought up. No one else in our family has *ever* stolen anything."

"It's not just thefts though, is it Tom?" He thrust the list before him then as he arched his eyebrows. "Criminal damage, burglary, graffiti, breaches." He whistled. "You've got a hell of a lot of convictions for someone so young."

"I'm gonna sort it out," Tom stated faintly.

"Course you are!" he laughed, snatching the sheet back towards him. "I see your type all the time! Little idiots that start off just like you are! You'll be inside by the time you're eighteen. Your sort never learn."

Tom reddened to the roots of his blond hair. I could tell he was rattled. For a moment I panicked that he might use an expletive from his collection but luckily, he didn't. That would have been a sure-fire way to have earned a little extra time in the cells! Grabbing the court summons, I muttered thanks to the man, and shepherded Tom towards the door.

Another Court Appearance (Lost Count Ages Ago)

"Theft of a bottle of beer to the value of £1.46! Theft of a dud firework!" The magistrate stared sceptically at us, and then at the people perched on the prosecution bench. "Is that it? What on earth is he doing before me?"

"Your honour," a woman from the bench sprang up like a jack-in-a-box. "He's got a substantial history of different types of thefts. It was deemed appropriate to prosecute for these, albeit more trivial acts of theft, as well."

The magistrate wiped his brow, almost knocking his glasses from the bridge of his nose in the process. Shaking his head, he addressed the clerk before him. "What is it you want me to do with him?"

"Your honour," began the duty solicitor, rising to his feet. "Tom deeply regrets his actions. He recognises that to steal these items was foolish, and indeed occasioned in what he has referred to as *moments of madness.*"

"Indeed," echoed the magistrate twisting towards where we stood. "Have you anything to say for yourself Thomas?"

"I just wanna say how sorry I am." Clasping his hands behind his back, he shuffled from one foot to the other. "It was stupid and I regret it."

"Regret you got caught you mean," barked the magistrate with a note of intolerance. "Not only are you a thief, it would seem that you're not actually a *good* one!"

I felt laughter bubbling within me as an image of Tom permeated my mind; the frustration that would have been upon his face as he attempted to ignite a fake firework!

"And you're his mother?" His gruff voice quickly quelled my emerging mirth. "How do *you* feel about him stealing?"

I started to get up.

"You may remain seated," he ordered. I compliantly dropped back into my seat with a thud.

"I am, of course, ashamed of him." I wrung my hands together, nervously. "And I can't believe we're here again."

"Quite," he agreed, drily, whispering something to the people poised at the bench in front of him.

"All rise." There was a rustle of clothing and a creaking of chairs in response to this order.

"Right Thomas," began the magistrate. "I've decided that in view of the value involved in this theft, I shan't impose any punishment on this occasion. It is however, imperative," he slapped the heel of his hand onto the desk, "that you continue to comply with the terms of your supervision order."

"I will, I promise," Tom nodded earnestly. "Definitely."

"If you are returned to this court for any more acts of theft, you must be aware that you *will* be leaving here in a prison van."

Tom nodded.

The judge then muttered something else to a clerk. "Court costs in this matter," he continued, averting his eyes towards me, "are payable by the defendants mother. Please collect the details on your way out."

Happy New Year

Tom

(16 years)

      Christmas had been shit! All I'd got was clothes and a crap phone. Me Mum had gone on one, big time, because I'd taken me mobile out of her room two days before Christmas. It's not as though I stole it or owt. I just had it a bit early. It was mine wasn't it? She went berserk as usual! I looked in Argos and it only cost fifty notes anyway.

Most of me mates got decent phones and gold chains and that, but not me. Their mums weren't tight like mine. It didn't even have a memory card so I could save me tunes. *What good's that?* She doesn't use hers anyway. It was a week before she even noticed I'd pinched it.

"What right have you got to take *my* memory card?" She was always fucking screaming.

"It's not as if you need it, is it?" *Well she didn't.*

"It's got all my photos on," she bawled, frothing at the mouth. "I want it back."

"It's not got em on any more." I turned to walk out of the room. *Oh shit, I'm gonna get it now!*

"You mean you've wiped it?" She was screeching as though she was in pain.

"Yeah, there weren't that many pictures on it anyway."

"How dare you?" *That bloody voice!* "All those pictures of the dog as a puppy, and Alex, and ......" *Yeah right. Precious dog. Precious Alex. That's all she bleeding cares about!*

Still, she picked me up after I'd been out new years' eve. Had been to an all-nighter. It was the bizz. Was still buzzing when her car pulled up. Could nearly block her out going on at me.

"What do you think you're doing reversing bloody charges again?" As usual, she was driving like an idiot. "You've put about twenty quid on our bill in the last few weeks! Where've you been anyway? It's half six in the morning. Don't you think I deserve a lie in new years day?"

And on, and on. In my head, I tried to replay one of the tunes from the club. Anything to drown the out drone of her voice. I should've charged up my phone so I could've plugged myself in to banging tunes, and not have had to endure her.

"You've bust the fridge-freezer, as well. Leaving the bloody door open all the time. I'd only just been shopping too. We've had to put it all in the shed. You don't give a toss do you?" And on she went.

I'd had enough of the lot of em if the truth be known. Which is probably why I got wrecked on Christmas day! I drank so much that mum left me with her brother! It was him who got me drunk anyway.

He fell out with me the morning after though. Caught me wearing one of his coats under mine. Well he's got loads a stuff hasn't he? It's not fair. Then he found the pouch of baccy I'd sneaked into the pocket as well.

They all had a right blast at me. Mum's said she won't take me to their house again. Am I bothered?

On Boxing day, I was dragged to a naff 'family' party. Some old dear that my grandad knows, who's eighty or summat. I wasn't complaining though. Posh house, nice grub and as much drink as you could hold.

Mum went barmy cos I filled my pockets up with a few bottles. Well what am I supposed to do when it's all free? I must have topped up from the night before cos I was soon wrecked again.

Spoiled a family photo! Sweet. Can't help it if I felt sick can I? Didn't get out of the shot in time. Mum looked like she was gonna die of embarrassment. Serves her right. She couldn't get me into the car quick enough.

"You're a disgrace!" Her anger making her even uglier than usual.

"All right Sarah, calm down." At least Martin was being reasonable for a change.

"And your language in that house was disgusting!" She whacked her hand against the steering wheel. "You sound as though you come from the gutter!"

"Shut the fuck up you weirdo!" I was starting to feel sick again. No wonder, having a mother like her. "Your voice goes right through me!"

"I can't wait to drop you off at your dad's." She turned to eyeball me, then twisted back to the road. "It's time *he* dealt with you. It's been ten months since you last slept there."

"It's not my fault if he doesn't want me!"

"It is. And I can't say I blame him either."

"That's just it, innit Mum? None of you want me." A wave of self pity washed away the wave of sickness. "I'd be better off dead."

"Oh shut up!" But the expression on her face showed I'd made her feel guilty. Sweet.

Luckily I made it to the bog when we got to his house. Only just though.

"Thanks a bunch!" I could hear my dad's voice in between my retching. "How the hell's he got into that state?"

"How do you think? He's all yours anyway. I need a break. If only for one night."

She left straightaway. Normally she'd have stayed for a drink so she could slag me off to Elizabeth. Seemed like she couldn't get out fast enough.

I slumped next to my dad, still feeling pretty dodgy.

"You stink!" was about the only conversation he was offering.

"Chill Dad." I slapped his arm. "I'll be gone tomorrow."

I thought I'd got rid of the silly cow but ten minutes later, I could hear her voice screeching down the phone to my dad.

"Right OK. I'll ask him. Yep. We'll check. Right, we'll have a look. I'll ring you back in a bit." A man of many words is my dad.

"Right mate." He turned to me. "Your mum's pretty upset."

"She always is." I raised my eyes to the ceiling.

"Apparently an expensive phone's disappeared from that birthday thing you were at." His face was fixed on mine.

"And she thinks it's me?" I leapt up from the sofa. "Well that's just fucking great innit! I get blamed for fucking everything!"

"Stop swearing Tom. That's gonna get you nowhere. Did you nick it or not?"

"No. Course I didn't. I've got a phone! Anyway, there's no point me even saying owt." I stormed towards the door. "Everyone'll blame me anyway! You needn't think I'm off home tomorrow. No way am I facing her, going on at me about it. It wasn't me!" I slammed up the stairs, away from the lot of em.

So that was it. Christmas and New Year. Another shitty year to look forward to. Me mates mostly had sound families. Not me though. I couldn't stand mine. I couldn't wait to get away from em. Especially my mother.

Letter from The Child and Adolescent Mental Health Team

7 January 2010

Dear Sarah,

We are writing to confirm that we are discharging Tom from our service as he has stopped attending the meetings with his counsellor. We hope this will not stop him accessing therapy in the future if he feels he would like to talk to someone. He would need to do this either via his gp or by accessing other young people's services.

We refer to our previous conversation when we confirmed that the conclusion of our assessment was that Tom did not have any underlying mental health diagnosis. It is our view that the emotional and behavioural difficulties Tom has presented with from an early age, reflects his experiences within the family system.*

We acknowledge this is difficult for you to hear without some sense of blame which we discussed with you previously, and our hope was that we could support you with thinking about this, in terms of how relationships develop within the family, how this impacts upon the children, and how you might respond to current difficulties within this context.

We know, Sarah, that you experienced a difficult early life history and childhood, and we feel that this has inevitably impacted on your relationship with Tom. We acknowledge it felt too difficult for you to engage with any work on this, which resulted in us focusing on individual work for Tom, and we offered him appointments accordingly.

Unfortunately we are unable to offer any further appointments as he has not attended on a consistent and regular basis. We hope things have improved and we wish you well for the future.

Yours sincerely

Child and Adolescent Mental Health Practitioner

*Blamed again.

Impossible

It was on days like this that I questioned how much longer I could go on.

5.41 am Awoken by doorbell. Tom collapses in door, looking like the living dead. Lie awake listening to him clattering around the kitchen as he reheats his meal cooked the previous evening.

9.05 am   Telephone call from youth offending team to inform me that he missed the appointment that he should have attended the day before. The court summons is on its way.

10.00 am   The post arrives. Huge phone bill caused by Tom ringing mobiles and making reverse charge calls. Warning letter due to non-attendance at last reparation session.

10.35 am   Tom starts moving around upstairs. Downstairs, we await his arrival on tenterhooks; preparing ourselves for the inevitable onslaught of his acidic tongue.

10.50 am   He literally throws Alex out of the chair he wishes to sit in, snatches the remote control, and sits down without a word to anyone. Told to fuck off when I try to reprimand him.

11.10 am   Whilst I make a drink, he grabs my lap top to log onto the internet. When I remind of the fact that it is only six weeks since I gave him my old lap top, he admits without remorse that he has sold it.

12.30 pm   We all feel instantly less on edge as the door bangs behind him. The entire house stinks of Lynx deodorant and the remains of his sullen anger.

12.42 pm   Martin discovers that Tom has stolen £10 from his wallet. A heated discussion ensues between the two of us.

3.35 pm   Tom appears in the kitchen, having stealthily entered through the back door. I interrupt him stuffing his pockets with as much 'convenience' food as possible. He is once again 'off his head.' I avoid confrontation.

7.45 pm   Without a word he barges past me as I stand in the doorway between our kitchen and living room. He opens the microwave door before slamming it shut. "Is that it?" he bellows.

"Do you expect me to scoff that muck?" Barely coherent, he is definitely in the grip of something he has taken.

7.55pm   I watch sadly as he takes his tray upstairs, preferring to eat alone in his room.

9.10pm   I put my head around his door to offer him a drink. He is asleep.

11.40pm   Engine revs outside our house. Driver repeatedly sounding horn. I open my window and angrily ask the grinning occupant of the car what he wants. He gives a one-word answer 'Tom.' Tom crashes around in his room for several minutes before heading downstairs to use a knife for operating the kitchen window lock.

Warrant for Arrest (*mine!*)

Magistrates Court

Division: 135

Case Number: 14099875463

A warrant has been issued in respect of the unpaid sum of £95.03, payable on behalf of Mr Thomas Clifford by his parent Mrs Sarah Pearson.
The above named has failed to pay the outstanding sum of £95.03, as ordered by the court, therefore this warrant is granted in order that further enforcement can commence.*
In order to prevent this arrest you can make full payment quoting the reference above to the Fines Officer.**
Failure to pay immediately will result in your arrest and/or imprisonment if default continues.
All enquiries regarding this warrant should be made directly to the court.

Acting Justices' Clerk

*I *had* stopped paying as a letter had been sent to Tom informing him that the debt had been cleared. I recall being annoyed at the time because a cheque had even been issued to *him* for £5, in respect of an overpayment *I* had made!
** I was told I had to make immediate payment by debit card. This was the only way I could prevent my arrest. Even though the aforementioned £5 cheque had been an administrative error, they would not back down and allow me more time.

Two Faced

February 2010 (16 years, 2 months)

As it was Martin's fortieth birthday, we had persuaded Elizabeth and Peter to have Tom for four nights, enabling us to go with Alex and the dog to a log cabin at the Lake District. Tom would have been bored rigid, had he accompanied us. In any case, our previous holiday experiences with him had put me off taking him along for eternity!

Even though I was ninety miles away from him, my handbag remained perched firmly on my shoulder and I fretted constantly about what he might be up to and with who. I was paranoid that he might break into our house whilst it was unoccupied or cause mayhem in our street with his mates. Sometimes, I speculated as to whether I would ever relax again.

Elizabeth updated me regularly. As it approached midnight on our second night of freedom, she informed me that he had not yet reappeared at their house. Knowing the buses would soon stop running, I began to panic. I had visions of him being in trouble or stranded somewhere. Yet obviously I was powerless to do anything!

She texted me soon after to say he had just arrived but with a massive gash on his cheek. He seemed drunk, stoned or whatever and had explained he had been in a fight and threatened with a broken glass. I didn't sleep that night; fearing his enemies would continue acting upon whatever vendetta they had with him.

The next morning, I received another text message. Tom needed stitches but was adamantly refusing to go to hospital. His story had now changed to the tune of he had fallen in the street onto some glass.

I was mortified when I got home. The injury had altered his handsome face, making him look thuggish.

Opinion of my Mother-In-Law
Divulged by Martin after telephone conversation with her

*"Well something must have made him like this!
Didn't Sarah show him enough love when he was younger?"*

Another Breach Charge, Another Court Appearance

The youth offending team had begun listing his court appearances on Fridays. His worker had gleaned that this was *my* day off; I could not be excused from attending with him. Some might say that at sixteen-years-old, he should be held accountable for his own actions. I would be inclined to agree. I would have to wait until he reached seventeen for that privilege though.

On this occasion he was being 'breached' yet again for non-compliance with his supervision and reparation orders. I had arranged to meet him outside the court.

I smelt Tom before seeing him as I meandered towards the formidable revolving court doorway. The security official recoiled when presented with the task of frisking him.

"You'll have to excuse him," I joked. "He must have been spraying testers in Boots. One day he'll learn that less is more!"

The two men did not flinch, smile, or offer any reply. Obviously someone of my calibre did not have the right to be conversing with them. Instead I choked, possibly on my own laughter but more probably on the overkill of aftershave. It made my eyes sting as we journeyed in the lift up to the youth court.

Once outside the courtroom, my mood darkened. Tom was stoned; very stoned indeed.

"Are you stupid or something?" I hissed, blushing as several pairs of ears tried to decipher our conversation.

A worker from the youth offending team skipped over to us.

"Don't worry Tom," she bristled, plonking herself beside him. "You're going to be fine in there. We'll be arguing for the court to keep an eye on your attendance for a month. They *should* leave it at that. So hopefully they won't be doing anything with you today."

"So he gets *no* form of punishment for blatantly defying his court orders." I spoke now, leaning forward in my seat so she could see me from beyond where Tom was slumped between us.

"We know how it is for him. At least he's honest." She patted his shoulder affectionately. "When he forgets; at least he admits he's forgotten. There's no inventing of elaborate excuses."

"He doesn't forget." I shook my head as I spoke. "He *chooses* not to attend, even though I remind him about all of his appointments."

She chose to ignore my comments. "We've all got a soft spot for Tom you know. It's obvious that there's a lovely lad lurking beneath all that bravado."

"Tom Clifford," trilled a girl who can't have been much older than he was. "Can we have five minutes before you go in?" She waved at him from the other side of the stark corridor.

Inquisitively I peered at her.

"Jennifer Phillips." She offered her hand. "Henry Hague Solicitors."

I shook the exquisitely manicured hand. "Have I to sit in with him?"

"Of course," she beckoned for us to follow her into the cramped interview room. On entering the windowless space, I was immediately swamped by the waft of sour sweat which must have lingered from the previous interviewee.

"Right." Her voice was shrill and highly pitched. "We're here today on charges of breach."

Tom shifted in his seat, looking as though he was struggling to keep his red-rimmed eyes ajar.

"Do you accept the charges Tom?" She shifted papers around in front of her.

"Yeah, I forgot about my appointments, that's all." He was barely audible.

"That's rubbish," I interrupted, trying to nudge him into alertness. "He chooses not to go. He's fully aware of his appointments."

"O-K." She gave me a curious look. "I think we'll keep that quiet in there.

I notice from these notes, that you've got a bit of a drug problem. Is that affecting your ability
to attend your appointments?"

"I smoke a bit of weed sometimes, that's all." He seemed to be slipping further down beside me. "But I haven't touched it for ages."

"He's talking even more garbage now!" I lifted my eyes towards the grotty ceiling. "He's stoned now! He smokes the stuff seven days a week!"

"Why are you doing this to yourself Tom?" Her voice was gentle.

"It's just my mates and that, innit."

She peered at me through her thickly rimmed glasses. "Is he getting any support with his drug problem?"

"We've tried." I sat up straight. "Support can only be given to a person who actually wants it. He seems to prefer this path. He knows there's an alternative."

"Don't chat shit Mum. I haven't touched weed for weeks."

"How can you sit there and say that?" I shrieked. "You're off your head now!"

His face reddened.

"How could you be so stupid?" I grabbed his arm. "Turning up here......stoned!"

"Can I speak to Tom alone?" The solicitor was commanding, rather than requesting, so I scuttled out of the room. She probably knew as well as I did that I was not the best person to be accompanying Tom to court. *How could I be on his side anymore? After all he had and was continuing to put us all through?*

Minutes later they emerged from the room. She indicated for me to follow them into court.

I obediently pottered behind as she lurched in on high heels. The magistrate signalled for everyone to sit apart from me and Tom.

"State your name," commanded someone from the bench.

"State your address."

"And you are accompanied by…" He glared at me over gold-rimmed spectacles.

"Sarah Pearson."

"You may sit," he beckoned to me. I dropped into my seat like a stone. "You stay standing," he ordered Tom.

The charges were read out; then the lady from the youth offending team was invited to speak. I listened attentively as she portrayed Tom as being amenable to work with; honest and committed to sorting himself out; just in with a 'bad' crowd.

The solicitor verified these comments, stating that Tom's main issue with attendance was the fact that his reparation order had to be executed on a Saturday morning. This, she stated, was bound to pose problems given the fact that he socialised on a Friday night.

Surely they're not going to find sympathy with that, I thought, bitterly.

"Remind me what this order was originally imposed for," demanded the magistrate, flicking through papers.

"You're honour." A lady on the prosecution bench sprang from her seat. "It was for an act of burglary and a further act of shoplifting occasioned in September of last year."

"I see." He rhythmically rubbed at his chin whilst appearing submerged in thought, before speaking in a low voice with his colleagues. He then cleared his throat and looked towards me.

"It would seem, Mrs Pearson; that an electronic tagging device might be the way forward here. Clearly Tom is struggling to comply with his orders, particularly the one that must be attended on a Saturday morning." He stretched his arms out, clasping his fingers together in front of him. "If we can ensure he is at home each evening; that would surely rectify that little problem."

"Am I allowed to disagree?" I stammered, feeling insignificant as my voice echoed around the courtroom.

"Well, yes, you are. It is, after all, *your* home where the equipment would be installed. But I cannot understand why you would *want* to disagree." He arched an eyebrow.

"Because, sir, electronic tagging has been tried on two occasions already." My voice wobbled into the air. "It has resulted in me having to endure a driveway full of hooded youths, smoking cannabis and making loads of noise while Tom leans out of his window or the front door to collude with them.

"I see."

"In addition, it makes family relations even worse than they already are. They are already stretched to breaking point."

"Would you care to elaborate on that?" He tipped his head to one side.

"Shut the fuck up Mum!" hissed Tom. From the look on his face, I knew the magistrate had heard him.

"You can glean from that little sentence, just how much respect he has for me." I was feeling a bit braver now. "You should hear him at home. The abuse I get's incredible." I took a sharp intake of breath before continuing. "I also have a younger son, who's eight. The example Tom sets is terrible; not to mention the bullying he has to endure."

"Stop fucking lying Mum," Tom elbowed me in the arm. "The court was eerily silent. They seemed intrigued by what I had to say.

"To have Tom at home each evening from 7pm again is unbearable as he has no respect whatsoever for any member of his family. He steals and verbally abuses us. His mates are just as nasty when they gather outside. Our neighbours don't even speak to our family anymore."

"What reason do you give for his behaviour?" One of the other magistrates spoke now.

"Drugs." The shame radiated from me as I imagined them struggling to make sense of this scenario in their sheltered existence. "He steals to fund his cannabis addiction. We've tried to get him help but he doesn't seem to want to stop.

"*Do* you want to stop Tom?" The first magistrate addressed him now.

"Yeah of course I do, but *she* just gets on my case all the time." He jabbed an accusing finger in my direction. "She never lets up."

"You wouldn't be the first teenager to say that about their mother," remarked the same magistrate, raising both eyebrows. "How about school? Do you enjoy school?"

"Yeah, I just wanna knuckle down and get good exam results," Tom asserted, possibly even convincing himself. "I wanna go in the army."

"Well, that's a commendable profession." All three magistrates appeared impressed. "Do you think you could assist him with enquiring into that, Mrs Pearson?

"Of course, but if he refuses to even go to school: then I don't see how he'll get into the Army." I shook my hair from my eyes. "He failed in mainstream school and has ended up at a pupil referral unit as it is.....look, I'm sorry to seem so negative," I continued, "but you don't know what I've been through. This must be the twentieth time I've been in this court. I've been his appropriate adult at the police station around the same number of times. I've had enough of it all. We're going round and round in circles.

"Have you *always* had problems with him?" The third, bespectacled magistrate spoke.

"Gosh, we're do I start. Put it this way, since he was two years old, I've dragged him to every specialist known to man. I've never had much help or a proper diagnosis though, hence we find ourselves where we are today."

I could sense the eyes of the youth offending woman boring into me. I addressed her directly.

"Look, I can imagine what you're thinking about me. You might believe the sun shines out of his backside. That's because he can talk the talk. What he can't do though is follow it through with any of what he promises. You'll all realise it sooner or later. You ought to try living with him. Try having to fit locks on all your doors and cart your handbag everywhere, even to the toilet!" My manic voice reverberated around the room. "I can't even leave Tom unattended with my younger son. And you should hear the abuse I endure each day because I won't give into his demands for money.

"We're not judging you." The youth worker's voice was gentle. "We're all aware you're in an intolerable position."

"We'll retire for several minutes," announced bespectacled. "We need to consider this carefully." The three magistrates rose from their chairs and filed out after one another.

"You stupid cow," Tom looked thunder at me. "I'm gonna get sent down cos of you. Why couldn't you just let em tag me?"

"Because I couldn't stand it again! No way! If they do send you down, it's *your* fault, not mine. It's *you* who breaks the law. *You* who commits the crimes." I rammed my finger towards him as I spoke. "You think you don't have to do the punishment though. You've had every bloody chance to sort yourself out!"

The rest of the room was silent. I realised they were probably all appraising me as a mother. Blaming *me* for his behaviour. Feeling sorry for *him*.

The five minutes seemed more like an hour. I began to fret that my words might be responsible for a custodial sentence. After all, this was about the eighth time he was before them on breach charges. Surely there was only so many times he could be let off for it?

My heart lurched uncomfortably as the three re-entered the courtroom. Everyone stood obediently. One of the magistrates smiled towards me. *Why is she smiling?* Perhaps I was about to be granted respite? Or maybe she thought I would be relieved that he was about to be given another chance?

It turned out to be the latter. He was given further hours of reparation to do and another 'stern' warning.

"We'll be maintaining an close eye on you. A note will be made on your file. You *really* are on your final chance. *Any* more charges, *any* more breaches, you'll be dragged back in front of us, personally. Do you understand?"

"Yes," Tom nodded furiously.

"So if there *is* a next time, bring an overnight bag with you, as you'll be needing it."

Doe anyone Ever Listen?

"Is that Tom's mum?" I didn't recognise the voice.
"Yes."
"It's Mr Johnson, head of the learning centre speaking. I'm ringing to let you know Tom's not feeling too well."

It was Monday morning. Tom had hardly been at home all weekend apart from Sunday. He had come in at noon and slept for most of the remainder of the day. Clearly he had overdone whatever substances he had been inflicting upon himself. I relayed this to the 'head of centre.'

"I believe he's genuinely ill, Mrs Pearson. He doesn't look too good at all."

"Well hopefully he'll keep in mind how rough he's feeling, and decide against the same course of action *next* weekend."

"We're going to have to request that you come and collect him."

"*I'm* not collecting him!" My voice rose up. "If you can't have him in school then he'll have to make his own way back on the bus."

"He doesn't look well enough for that."

"Look, I'm not being rude, but his *illness* is self-inflicted. I'm afraid I haven't got a
shred of sympathy for him."

"But we have your authorisation to release him from the centre?"

"Yes. I'm surprised even he's bothered about permission," I snorted. "Normally he'd just find a way out when he wants to leave."

"Like I said, Mrs Pearson, I don't think he's well enough for that."

It was several hours before Tom made an appearance at home. He stumbled in, stoned, turned out the kitchen cupboards onto a tray then spent the rest of the evening, sated, in his room.

The next morning after I had succeeded in packing him off towards the bus stop I decided to ring his school.

"I'm just calling to inform you that Tom's on his way."

"Oh, is he feeling better now?"

"There was nothing wrong with him, just as I'd suspected. After he'd been allowed to leave school yesterday, he passed the rest of the day getting wasted with his mates."

"Right……I'll let Mr Johnson know."

"If you could. Tom is usually below par on a Monday, but it's only because of what he does to himself over the weekend."

"We'll bear that in mind in future, thanks."

"I did try to tell this to Mr Johnson yesterday but it would appear that Tom put on a convincing performance.

"This message is for Tom's Mum." It was the following Monday. *"This is Mr Johnson speaking, head of the learning centre. Just a message to let you know that Tom's on his way home. He's got earache."*

My hollow laugh echoed around the silence of the kitchen, bouncing like missiles off the walls. *Was this man an idiot or what?*

<u>Here is a message I *could* have left in response</u>

This message is for Mr Johnson. This is Tom's Mum speaking. Just a message to let you know that Tom came straight home; after being despatched from school with 'earache.' As I have recently highlighted, Tom is addicted to cannabis and possibly other substances. He suffers the after effects at their worst on a Monday after the excesses of the weekend. However, he seems perfectly OK today and is certainly well enough to bully me for money. Thanks to him not being in school, I have spent the afternoon enduring the company of his associates outside my house. No doubt their language, general conduct, engine revving and drug smoking has been duly noted by my neighbours.

I wonder if you could clarify why you haven't paid any attention to the comments I made a week ago – do you think you know Tom better than I do?

Quote from Alex

"He stays out all night and sleeps all day. He's just like a bat Mummy."

More than Cannabis

April 2010 (16 years, 4 months)

"Oh no!" I exclaimed as I flung the door open to two policewomen.

"It's OK, it's positive news for a change!"

"Oh?" This I was definitely interested in hearing!

"There was some trouble in the town centre last night, brawling, that sort of thing. Tom stayed out of it, even though we lifted several of his mates. We were impressed with him actually. As we were passing by your house anyway, we decided to give you better news for once."

"Thanks for that." My tension drained from me like fat from a pricked sausage. It certainly makes a pleasant change to hear something positive. I was happy but at the same time, irked, by the three sets of net curtains trembling enquiringly from across the road.

"He's mixing with a dire crowd though," asserted the other officer, her smile fading to a frown. "They'll drag him down with them if he's not careful, you know."

"We do know about his friends." Folding my arms, I propped myself against the frame of the doorway. "Which is why we don't allow *any* of them in the house. We've tried to talk to Tom, but at the end of the day ...."

"I know.........it's hard...... but perhaps him staying out of last night's fracard is a sign he's turning the corner."

He didn't return home that night. If he had I would have praised him to the skies for staying out of the trouble that had occurred. It was 8.30 the next morning, before he surfaced, looking as though he had not slept for weeks.

"Thanks for ringing to let me know where you were." I surveyed his scrawny form. The weight was tumbling from him. "Don't you think you should get ready for reparation?"

"I came to ask for some money." His eyes implored me. "For bus fare and something to eat."

I thrust a note at him, then watched as he swaggered down the garden path to his friend who was waiting on the wall, hiding behind a hood.

"I bet he's not going," Martin stated, wrinkling his face up.

"Don't be daft, he wouldn't be that stupid."

Later that afternoon, as I relaxed with my book, my heart plunged towards my stomach as I noticed a familiar, yet unwelcome police van drawing up outside our house. Martin and I pounced on the door handle in unison.

"I'm afraid it's not such good news today," the police officer informed us as we stood before her. "Is he in?"

"No, I've not seen him since this morning. What's he done now?"

"We've been called out to investigate a noise complaint. When the occupants answered the door, we smelt drugs. So we went in and managed to seize a substantial quantity."

"From Tom?"

"No. As we entered, he leapt from a window. Which makes him look pretty suspicious." Her gloved hands held a bag of white powder aloft. "If his prints are on these, he's in trouble."*

Tom seemed done in when he returned that evening. It was the worst state I had ever seen him in. His eyes were raw, his skin blotchy and his lips swollen. But it was his nose that worried me most. It was misshapen; as though he had been hit, it even appeared to have moved slightly. His clothes draped from him as though he were a clothes hanger. He looked ill, very ill.

"Look at the state of you," I shrieked, grabbing hold of his shoulders to take a closer look at him. "What on earth have you taken?"

He mumbled incoherently, exuding the air of a down-and-out instead of a healthy sixteen-year-old, with his entire life before him. After he had staggered up to bed, I slunk onto the sofa and rested my head in my hands.

"That isn't drink," Martin stated softly, landing beside me. "I couldn't even smell it on him, could you? Did you see the state of his eyes? And his nose? God knows what he's been on."

"I know. Fighting my tears, I lifted my head. "He looks terrible. What're we going to do?"

All through the night I was kept awake by Tom snortingas he tried to clear his nose. It was late afternoon when his haggard body finally surfaced. By then he had slept for nearly twenty four hours.

*We didn't hear anything further in relation to the confiscated white powder. Tom explained how he had jumped from the window in a panic, assuming he would be blamed. Hmmmm.

Trying to Get Through

"Is this *really* how you want to be spending your life?" I was worried sick about him. Obviously unable to face it, he had pushed his Sunday roast away. It was one of his favourite meals usually. "Tom, you're a young lad." My knife and fork clattered onto the table. "You're either in some sort of trance, or you're asleep or ill. What're you doing to yourself?"

Suddenly he looked upset. "I don't know. I want to sort it out Mum. Honest, I do."

"Then why don't you?" From across the table, I rested my hand on his. "You're not on your own for God's sake. You've got us. We'll do anything to help you, you know."

"You're sounding pretty sorry for yourself Tom." Martin was more abrupt than me. "Are you sure it's just drugs? Or perhaps you've done something else you regret this weekend?" He continued shovelling dinner into his mouth without looking at Tom.

"Why do you always have to think the worst of me?" Tom sipped at his water, head bowed.

"Experience."

"Next weekend," I began, trying to steer them from confrontation, "why don't you do something with *us*? Remove yourself from the temptation of your mates." Jumping up, I then began stacking plates as I tried to persuade him. "I know we can be a bit boring but you could choose what we do. The cinema, bowling, something to eat, anything."

"I will," he agreed, twisting himself around in his seat to face me as I started filling the sink. "I want to get away from that crowd anyway. Make some decent mates."

"Talking the talk again Tom?"

I glared at Martin as he spoke between mouthfuls. It was time to change the subject.

"Have you spoken to anyone from 'careers' at school yet? Once I know what you want to do, I could get you some forms organised for college?"

"I'll ask tomorrow." Absently, he drove the salt and pepper pots around the table.

"You could have the world at your feet, if only you'd sort yourself out." Pausing my bashing around of pans. I looked at him. "I'm so worried about you."

"There's no need. Chill Mum"

"Oh come on, you don't bother to come home half the time. You don't even ring me to let me know where you are."

"I've not got a phone anymore," he avoided my eyes.

"But you've only had it five minutes!" I wiped my hands on a tea towel.

"I flogged it."

"How much?" Martin slammed his cutlery onto his plate.

"I should never have listened to you!" I glared at Martin. "It was you who went on at me to get him another phone! I knew he'd sell it." I marched from the sink and flung myself back down onto the dining chair. Go on then Tom, how much?"

"Thirty quid."

"*Thirty quid.* But it cost bloody eighty!"

More Sleepless Nights

"Mummy." I sat up, responding to Alex's tapping on my bedroom door.

"Hang on sweetheart." Rubbing the sleep from my eyes, I navigated my way around the bed in the darkness.

"I can't sleep again. I've been laid awake for ages. Can I get up for a bit?"

I glanced towards the clock which glowed across the room. 3:26 am. "Alex, it's the middle of the night." I clutched his hand. "You must try and get back to sleep."

"But I can't." He padded at the side of me back to his room. "I keep hearing things."

"Like what?"

"Someone outside." As he clambered back into bed, he pointed towards his window.

"There's no one outside." Peeking through his curtains, I shook my head at him.

"Has Tom come home?"

"No, not yet." My heart sank at this reminder. It would take me ages to get back off to sleep now.

"So even if I *do* get to sleep, he'll only wake me up with the doorbell anyway." Tears filled his eyes as he remained sat upright in his bed. "I want to go to sleep Mummy but I can't."

I stayed with him whilst he had a drink, before tucking him back up and leaving him. Within an hour he was rapping at my door again.

"Oh bloody hell!" moaned Martin, tugging a pillow over his head. "It's the third night in a row he's been like this!"

"It's not his fault!" I sprang back up again. "It's no wonder he's so unsettled with everything he has to contend with!"

"Well go and see to him then!"

Alex's bottom lip trembled as I opened the door to him. "Come on, it's OK, I'll take you back to bed." I reached for his hand. "Don't listen to daddy, he's just grumpy."

The next day I stocked up with lavender spray, hot chocolate and a CD of *calming classical music for children.* None of it worked though. Meanwhile, in the days that followed, Alex was working himself up into more and more of a state.

"I'm scared of it being night time," he would plead. "I'm so worried I won't be able to sleep again." His eyes were dark against his pale skin.

"You will, I promise."

"I can't stop worrying about it. It's making my head hurt."

"Alex," I drew him towards me and looked directly into his face. "Every time you get the worry in your mind, you must try to chase it away by thinking about something happy."

"Like what?" He frowned. "We're not even going on holiday this year, are we? We can never do anything because of *Tom*."

"We'll still do nice things, you'll see. We can go for trips out for the day or you can have a friend round, or……"

"I can't have a friend round. Not with Tom." His voice trembled. "He'll be mean to them like he is to me."

Alex's sleeplessness continued for well over a fortnight. He worked himself into an incredible turmoil about it. Usually, other than his asthma, he never caused me any worry. But I was on the verge of consulting a doctor as he looked exhausted.

Then miraculously, one night, he slept for the entire night without waking. We were all elated. Then he slept the next night and the next. Guilt consumed me though. I had always endeavoured to shield him from the anxiety that we, as grown ups, suffered. But it was evidently not possible.

Arrested Again

Martin

It was the middle of the day but I needed to lie down with a blistering headache. Tom and Alex were at school, Sarah was working and the dog was slumbering in her basket in the kitchen. As I reclined in the tranquillity of the house, the pressure in my head began to subside.

BANG! BANG! BANG! I was jolted into life. The dog was barking hysterically at whoever pounded upon the door. BANG! BANG! BANG! BANG! BANG! She began to growl. Then the thumping became apparent on the back door too. Too in pain to move, I just listened. BANG! BANG! BANG! It persisted for at least five minutes. Whatever it was, I couldn't face it now.

The hum of several deep voices was drowned in the din of an engine being fired up. Vehicle doors slammed as an engine revved. *I had to know who it was!* In order that the occupants of the vehicle didn't see me, carefully I peered around the side of the curtain, recoiling at the enormous police van, normally deployed for riot purposes. *What on earth had Tom done now?*

Later that afternoon, I seized the opportunity to quiz him before Sarah arrived home.

"I don't know what they want me for," he protested, slinging his coat across the sofa. "Maybe it's that drugs thing from that party last Saturday." Contemplating the situation aloud, he began preparing a snack. I listened intently. "Or it could be about some graffiti. Me and me mate nicked some spray cans. But we cleaned it off like."

"I can't see the police sending a riot van for that Tom!" I passed him the margarine from the fridge.

"The only other thing it might be is that me mates nicked a couple of boats from the side of the lake. It was the other day when I was at school. They just took em out for a laugh and that. It was nowt to do with me though." His eyes met mine as though he was searching for belief.

"Well if that's the case, your mother will ring school and they'll confirm when you were there, and let the police know." I headed for the door. "If you've done nothing wrong then there's no need to worry."

"I haven't. And if anyone says I have, they're lying."

Knotted up Inside

I could not sleep yet again that night. *What had Tom done?* The police would not disclose a thing when I rang to ask. They would only say that they were intending to return the following day to arrest him. If I failed to ensure he was 'available,' they had threatened to return in the middle of the night.

It was after three the next afternoon when the riot van reappeared. How I had kept him in the house all day, I will never know.

"I am arresting you on suspicion of car theft and street robbery," asserted a plain-clothed man who had introduced himself as CID something or other. "You have the right to remain silent, etc, etc."

"Street robbery!" I gasped, sinking onto the stairs.

"Whoever's saying I was there is making it up!" Tom, however, compliantly allowed the men to handcuff him.

"Come on lad, we'll discuss it down at the station." Two of the uniformed officers led him down my drive towards their van. I quelled the urge to rebelliously wave at our neighbouring observers!

The plain-clothed 'CID' hung back to search our house.

"Will this take long?" I sighed. "I've to collect my eight-year-old from school shortly."

Later that evening I had to attend the police station in my capacity as 'appropriate adult.' Tom had opted for a solicitor. We had a brief discussion before the commencement of the interview.

"I'm not naming any names," Tom stated adamantly, resting his elbows on the graffiti-covered table.

"That's fine," nodded the solicitor, scribbling onto a notepad. "Just tell them you're fearful of repercussions. You can also, as I'm sure you're aware, say *no comment* at any time."

Moments later, two CID men entered the airless interview room. One of them was the man who had searched our house earlier. The other I recognised, but could not place.

"Don't I know you," he looked at me searchingly as he sat down, his chair jarring against the hard floor.

God, where do I know you from? It was agonising! *Please let it not be an embarrassing acquaintance!*

"Ah yes, I remember; this isn't the first time we've met Tom, is it?" A flicker of recognition crossed his face. "I seem to recall arresting him for burgling your next-door-neighbour some years ago."

"Two years."

The solicitor shuffled uncomfortably in his seat.

"Right, let's get started." The other officer began unwrapping the tapes.

There was a pause as a long tone sounded on the tape recorder, signalling that the interview was commencing. We all had to state our names; Tom was again read his rights then asked if he understood what he had been arrested for.

"It wasn't me," he protested, leaning back in his chair. "I know who it was and it wasn't me. I shouldn't even be here."

"Let's deal with this one thing at a time." One of the CIDs asked the questions while the second transcribed the conversation onto an A4 pad. His handwriting looked like spiders venting their anger all over the page. "Firstly the street robbery. Describe to me, in your own words, exactly what happened on the evening of last Friday, 25th April."

Tom drew a deep breath in. "I was at a party yeah, and a few of the lads decided to go out for a bit and they came back with this bag yeah, but I wasn't with em."

"Let's go back a bit." The CID formed a backwards gesture with his hands. "Who was at the party?"

Tom looked reminiscent. "There was a few lasses, me and three other lads."

"Names?" The second CID spoke now with his pen poised.

"I don't know any of the lasses second names. And I only know two of the lads."

As Tom reeled off the names of the 'partygoers,' the second CID furiously scribbled them down.' *So much for him not being willing to name names!*

"What about the other lad?"

"I don't know his name."

"Can you describe him for us?" The first CID leaned forward in his chair.

"Well he looks a bit like me really. Blonde hair, nearly 6 foot."

"What sort of build is he?"

"I dunno."

The officer read out a description. "White male with blonde hair. Aged between 15 and 17. Wearing dark blue jeans, a light blue shirt and black trainers. Athletic build."

"Yeah that's right," Tom affirmed, nodded and raising his eyes to make contact with theirs. "That's what he looks like."

"Don't you think he sounds a lot like you?" Tom squirmed beneath four sets of probing stares. This line of questioning was pursued for a while but it soon became apparent that Tom was not budging. No way was he admitting to anything, just that the 'character,' as he dubbed him, had been a 'mentalist,' hurling verbal abuse at people in the street, kicking bins over and making strange suggestions about what they might do to obtain some money.

"How are you aware of all this, if you stayed at the house when it was all going on?" The CID sat back in his seat and clasped his hands behind his head.

"Cos one of me mates told me." Tom cocked his head, defiantly.

"Did you handle any of the stolen property?"

"No." He shifted in his seat.

"Could your fingerprints be on any of the stolen property?"

"No."

"Was it *you* who punched the victim in the face?"

Tom glanced at his solicitor. "No comment."

Tom was then asked a series of further questions, all requiring a 'yes' or 'no' response. To which he replied "*no comment.*" To all of them.

The other CID then shifted the focus onto the car theft. He stated the approximate time that it had occurred.

"Where were you on Monday morning between one and five am?" His voice sounded robotic.

I let out a jagged breath, momentarily feeling as though I was embroiled in a TV drama.

"In bed."

"Can you verify this?" All eyes flickered to me.

"*As far as I know* he was in bed. But I can't be sure. He climbs in and out of windows through the night."

"Shut up Mum," Tom glared towards me.

"Don't talk to your mother like that."

After thirty nine minutes, the interview was concluded. Tom was informed that he would be expected to participate in an ID parade. If the victim picked him out, it would be necessary to re-interview him.

It was a filmed ID parade. Like in all sombre situations, I suddenly felt an inappropriate burst of mirth which I mercifully stifled!

"Right Tom, I want you to select a t-shirt to wear," trilled the man conducting the filming. He was a cheery, bumbling man, with a humongous red nose and a beer belly. "I'd advise choosing a light coloured one if I was you." Half a dozen t-shirts in assorted colours were spread on the table in front of us.

"Why?" Tom started rummaging through them.

"Because," the man fiddled with his computer, "the description that's been given of the suspect, describes a lad wearing a *dark* t-shirt, that's all."

"Oh." Tom whipped off his own t-shirt and tugged a pale green one over his head. It was a colour he would never dream of wearing but it suited him anyway.

"Good," smiled the man, manoeuvring Tom onto a 'spot' in the centre of the room. "Now, I want you to look that way towards the camera and then back the other way. Keep your face straight and your hands by your sides."

Tom, with the scar emblazoned centrally upon his cheek, looked every inch the yob as he was captured on film.

"OK." He gestured for us to join him at the computer. "We'll slide your picture in with some others. I want you to pick another eight lads from these photos." He pointed at the screen. "Choose images with a similarity to yourself."

After they had all been decided upon, we reviewed the 'parade.' I have to say, he looked right at home amongst the other 'suspects'!

By this time he had been held in custody for six hours. I expected them to release him.

"Do you think he's telling the truth?" One of the officers looked at me. Shaking my head, I hardly dared to say the word out loud. Although I felt guilty about it, I could not lie.

"We don't believe a word," agreed the CID man. "But if he isn't picked out from the line up tomorrow, I'm afraid we have no evidence to place him at the crime. We'll keep him here tonight anyway."

"All night?" His words stung like a slap. Although I knew Tom was probably in it up to his chin, it didn't stop me fretting about his state of mind. I felt dreadful leaving him. Especially after the occasion when he had repeatedly thrown his head against the cell wall. Maybe I should have relaxed though. At least I knew where he was for a change! Nevertheless, I still endured a sleepless night!

The following day, I could not face going to work. My insides felt too churned up. The thought of my son, along with two of his 'friends,' cornering, attacking and mugging a defenceless, lone boy gnawed away at me. *How desperate must he be for money?*

To distract myself from my miserable thoughts, I drove to the supermarket, but just trudged around, unable to focus, probably doubling the time the shopping would have normally taken. At the checkout, I queued behind a woman and a teenage lad, who must have been about Tom's age. It became necessary to blink back tears as I observed them loading shopping onto the conveyor belt like it was the most normal thing in the world for a son to help his mother with the shopping.

An image of Tom, sitting alone in a cell, where he had been held since this time yesterday, refused to leave my mind.

That afternoon at four, he was released without charge, having spent nearly twenty four hours locked up. He had not been chosen from the line up, so returned home, jubilant.

"He's guilty as sin," Martin observed. "If I'd been locked up all this time for something I hadn't done, I'd be fuming! In fact I'd be suing the police for wrongful arrest! Tom just seems relieved that he's got away with it! Again."

Leaving School

Tom was approaching his final days at school. I attended a parent consultation evening. No progress had been made in terms of what he might do beyond school. In my opinion, he was in grave danger of aimlessly drifting deeper into his cesspit of inappropriate friends and criminal behaviour.

His English teacher and a 'key worker,' however, were enthusiastic about his drawing talent.

"If only he would develop it," she insisted, facing me in the barren classroom. "But he has no concentration skills whatsoever. He continually disrupts the others."

"No change there then."

"What do you mean?" She folded her arms.

"I've been having this conversation with his teachers for years. He's *always* been disruptive and unable to concentrate."

"Was he ever diagnosed with anything?"

"I've had him to a multitude of so-called specialists over the years. The closest I got to a diagnosis is when he was eleven and was identified as having a 'conduct disorder'.

"*We* haven't been made aware of any problems before high school." She glanced sideward's at her colleague.

I laughed. "I can't believe the lack of cohesion between services. No one talks to each other. I've had serious problems with him since babyhood. I've begged for help. I never got it. That's why we're still in this situation now!"

"Well. there's nothing on his file." She flicked through it as though something would suddenly leap out at her.

I shook my head. What could I say? It was clear they wanted insight but I did not have the energy to rake over our history yet again. The future was all I was interested in discussing now.

Eventually, we concluded that with my help, Tom would receive as much support as he would accept, to do his best in his forthcoming exams. The pupil referral unit would also seek careers advice and information about art college.

This, like many promises, failed to materialise. Ultimately, it was left to me to obtain careers advice and apply to college on his behalf. With four exams looming, he officially left the pupil referral unit. I obtained revision materials and attempted to gain interest from him. Unfortunately, I was unable to persuade him to do a stroke of work towards them.

Morning Calls

The situation at home was escalating further out of control. Each time Tom came home he seemed to be 'off his head.' It is the only way I can describe it.

At times he would disturb us just an hour after we had gone to bed; sometimes in the middle of the night; at other times it would be at dawn: at about four or five in the morning. I am not sure he had any concept of time. Increasingly, I came to suspected that he had progressed beyond cannabis in his drug use. His dependence seemed to lie in the snorting of mephedrone, or M-Cat, as it had been dubbed. It was terrifying for me.

Early one morning, when he hadn't been home all night, we were awoken by Tom and his 'friends' at the side of our house. It was 5.21 am. Martin headed to the landing window to observe their activity.

"They're measuring out white powder!" he exclaimed, hiding inconspicuously behind the curtain. "We should get the police here."

"They'd have moved before they got here. Look how long they've been in the past."

"Maybe I should get photos then," Martin suggested.

"And what if they see you?" I leaned back against my pillows. "Don't bother for God's sake! I don't want my windows going through!"

When confronted later that day with his early morning escapades, Tom shrugged casually and promised it would not happen again. He then loaded his pockets with food before disappearing. Later that evening he came home in a right state.

"Oh my God!" I grasped at his shoulders. "Your lips look as though they've been stung by a wasp." His nose was swollen too.

"Leave me the fuck alone!" He wrenched himself out of my grip and stamped up the stairs.

It was 5.32 the following morning when we were awoken again by the local thugs.

"Tom you dirty bastard!" Leering and whistles ensued, then several bangs as stones were lobbed at his window, bouncing off the glass.

I lay, frozen to the spot with my hand resting on the dog's back to try to stop her from growling. There was no point confronting the people outside – it wasn't worth the abuse. But my next door neighbour risked it. It was actually the first time she had.

"Go away and wake someone else up!" She cried wearily from her window. It was a fair request.

"Fuck off silly bastard!" was the response she received for her efforts. *Oh God, please don't let this get out of hand!*

"Go away little boy!"

"I'll put your fucking windows through!" It was a different voice now. I guessed there was at least four of them out there.

There then followed several laughs, sneers and a few more whistles before they seemed to disperse. Martin was swiftly dressing, poised to confront them if they returned. There was no point trying to go back to sleep. We were far too wound up.

Later that morning the man from next door pounded on our door. Tom was still asleep.

"I want names," he commanded in a trembling voice, his entire body shaking too.

Martin joined me at the door and reeled off three names of youths he had recognised that morning.

"Just so I know who I'm dealing with when my windows go through." The neighbour glared at me, accusingly.

"I'm so sorry. If there was anything I could be doing about the situation, I'd be doing it. I've confronted these idiots myself and been met with the same abuse as your wife."

"She's terrified," he continued. "We've three kids to consider you know."

"I do know. And if they turn up again I'll call the police. I'll have a word with Tom too, for all the good it'll do."

These were obviously not satisfactory enough responses for him. But I was sure he would sense my lack of control in who decided to cause trouble in our street.

"We're on the same side as you." I persisted. "Obviously, I want them all stopping as well."

"The thing is though, we've got one of the idiots living here!" Martin gestured up to Tom's window. "But if I had *my* way, he wouldn't be!"

"I'm trying to sort something out," I added. "*I* want him in his own place too. Then maybe the problems will ease a bit around here. All those other hoodies would have no excuse to keep hanging around. I'm just so sorry that it's impacted on other neighbours. It isn't fair on you and I'll do whatever I can to put a stop to it."

I spent all that day with a blistering headache, probably due to lack of sleep. Tom ventured out and returned in an even worse condition than the day before.

"What's up with you?" Martin glanced from his newspaper as Tom staggered into the living room.

"Feel like shit." He was clutching his stomach.

"Been on that stuff again, have you?"

"It's the last time." He sank weakly into an armchair.

"That's what you promised a couple of weeks ago."

"I mean it this time. I'm never feeling like this again." He was bent double.

"Is it that Mephedrone?" My brother Chris, over for dinner, spoke from behind the computer.

I nodded.

"It's serious shit, that, you know. It's wiping people out. Haven't you heard?"

Tom sat back up again. "I feel like my nose is caving in inside."

Chris continued. "I've heard it's as addictive as heroin. It's cut with other stuff too so you don't even know what you're snorting."

"How *are* you feeling, *exactly?*" I peered at Tom anxiously. You hear all sorts of horrific scenarios of teenagers on drugs; sudden heart attacks, fits, internal bleeding........

"I'm aching everywhere," he groaned. My head and nose are killing. I'm gonna have no nose left and it'll cost a few grand for a new one."

I shot Chris a harsh look as he stifled a chuckle.

"I feel like I'm gonna have heart attack or something." He lifted a hand to his chest. "My heart's beating really fast."

"When was the last time you ate?" I'd thrown his uneaten meals away for the previous two nights.

He shrugged.

"I've saved you some dinner." I started towards the kitchen. "I think you should try and eat a bit, then have a lay down upstairs. You might feel better after a bit of rest."

Picking at the food I placed before him, he seemed agitated.

"Would you say you've taken much of it Tom?" I flopped onto the chair beside him.

"They're all at it. Round at a house. And now I can't stop."

"How do you afford it? I thought drugs were expensive."

"Not Mephedrone." He pushed food around his plate as he spoke. "You can get it for the same price as a pack of fags."

"D'you think you're addicted to it?"

"I think so. I can't stop it anyway. Not now."

"I think I'd better make an appointment at the doctors. Maybe we can get you admitted into a clinic or something?" I would have robbed a bank at that moment to cover the cost.

"No it's not that bad. Look, Mum, I'm gonna sort it out, I'm gonna change, I promise you."

I put my hand on his arm as he struggled on with his meal.

"I'll help you. We'll discuss this more tomorrow when you've calmed down a bit. For now, though, I'm off to bed." I pushed my chair pack and stood up. "I've been up since half five. Get some rest Tom. Put your TV on and try to relax. You'll be OK, I promise. You just need to get this poison out of your system.

"I know."

I went to bed. But exhausted as I was, I couldn't settle. I slept fitfully, abruptly waking from a dozing state every so often with feelings of dread.

The next morning I did a bit more research about Mephedrone. All the symptoms he had been suffering from the previous evening were listed. I was worried to read that users become psychologically dependant on it. Furthermore, its use had been implicated in several heart attacks. It was classed as a 'narcotic' substance, a progression 'up' from cannabis, heading towards the 'biggies' like heroin and crack.

By eleven o'clock that morning, I was starting to panic. There had not been a sound from Tom's room. The fact that he was not yet out of bed was usual. But normally his bedsprings would creak as he moved. Or we would hear him lumbering to the toilet. Because I had not even heard him cough, I voiced my concerns to Martin.

"Go and see if he's alright then." He switched the lawnmower off.

"I can't. I'm scared." I kicked the grass he had mown into a pile.

"Of what?"

"He said last night that he felt like he was dying. What if he has?" Tears leapt to my eyes.

"Don't be so ridiculous! You're being daft. I'll go and give him a shout."

Relief washed over me when I heard Tom moaning at being woken up. It was at that moment that I reached a decision. Until I was convinced that he was not going to be tempted by any sort of drugs, he was getting no more money. Not from me, anyway.

This decision was further compounded when the post clattered on the mat:

4 June 2010

Dear Tenants,

Re: Nuisance to Neighbours

I have received a complaint with regard to your conduct towards one of our tenants.

The complaint is:
Youths congregating outside your house in the early hours of the morning shouting up to your son's bedroom window.

I would inform you that this department takes incidents of nuisance to neighbours and anti-social behaviour seriously and is determined to take steps to prevent them from being repeated and this may include taking legal action.

I would like to give you the opportunity to discuss the complaint and I would ask you to contact me as soon as possible. We can then agree how the matter can be rectified to ensure that no further complaints are made against you.

Yours sincerely

Housing Officer

I listened as Martin made the call. He was informed that someone more senior would call him back. *We were going to get thrown out! Where would we go? What the hell would we do?* All because of Tom.

Coming to a Head

The next evening Tom returned downstairs after we had all gone to bed. I lay, staring into the darkness, knowing I would get no peace until I discovered what he was up to. As I tiptoed down the stairs to investigate, I was greeted by the familiar herbal stink.

Before I could yell at him, I realised he had sneaked out of the kitchen window. It had been left ajar for his return, making our house vulnerable to whoever might be passing. I dashed to the front door, hoping he would still be in the vicinity but he had vanished into the night.

When he reappeared the next morning, I was already up. A vile mood radiated from him as he barged past me. Mercifully I did not have to remain in the house for long, as Alex was playing in a football tournament. I flinched as I packaged him into the car, trying to ignore the hate-filled insults that Tom was flinging at me from his bedroom window. His venom flooded the street.

"Slag!! Fucking tight bitch!" He bellowed into the Sunday morning calm. Obviously he was displeased at the fact that I hadn't left him any money!

As he launched something from his window at my car, I sped away. The meek and mild mood of the previous day had not lasted long.

A reasonably sympathetic 'senior housing officer' rang us back that morning, agreeing that we were unable to control the behaviour of *other* youths. But he warned Martin that if we did not begin to control *our* youth, we would definitely be facing eviction.

The man also made us aware that our neighbours were all maintaining a 'log' against *us*, whereby they were keeping track of any activity and adverse behaviour from Tom and his accomplices. *No wonder I was unable to hold my head up in the street.* All information was being reported back to the police, the housing office and the neighbourhood watch meetings. (Which of course *we* hadn't been invited to!)

As I had resolved, I refused to give Tom any money over the next few days. Reluctantly, I bought a stash of cigarettes and cans of pop to store in the house. I also bought pre-paid bus tickets. There was no way I was going to attempt another bus pass, so many had he lost!

I ferried him to several exams at the pupil referral unit, mainly to ensure that he definitely attended them. As we travelled together in the car, I attempted to encourage him to put together a portfolio for his forthcoming art college interview. I tried to discuss with him about how he was managing without mephedrone. However, the conversations were one-sided and he seemed subdued.

"I want some money," he stipulated after several days. His exams were over and he was clearly bored.

"Tom you know what I said." My stress levels were immediately elevated. *I had to stick to my resolution!*

"I only want bus fare."

"I'll give you a ticket." I began fishing around in my bag.

"What if I want cigs?"

"You can take some with you." I thrust a packet of cigarettes and a bus ticket towards him. He did not seem happy with the fact I had an answer for everything.

"Wouldn't it be worth a fiver just to get me out of your hair?"

"No."

"If you don't give me it, I'm going to annoy you until you do." He began whistling and tapping his feet. Ignoring him, I continued shuffling through paperwork.

"I mean it." His expression became more menacing. "I'm going to really get on your nerves."

"I'll just stay out of your way."

"Then I'll follow you around. C'mon Mum." He jumped up from his seat. "I need some money. Alright?"

Gathering my computer and my bits of paper, I decided to shut myself in my room. I had loads of work to do and was not going to give him the satisfaction of bullying me.

"I'm off upstairs." I began shuffling towards the door. "We've discussed this. You know why I'm not willing to give you money at the moment."

"Do that and I'll sit outside your room all day banging on your door." He manoeuvred himself behind me.

"Tom. You're not going to win this." I swung around to face him. "Back off."

His face darkened even more. "I fucking hate you, you stupid bitch." He took a step towards me. "Do you *know* how much I hate you?"

"I think you'd better go out." I backed away, noticing the hairs on the back of my neck rising to attention. I'm not sure whether it was fear or anger. Probably both.

"Fucking whore," he persisted. "Tight fucking whore."

That was it. My temper was starting to erupt. I dumped the computer and papers back onto the table.

"Get out of my house," I pleaded, tugging at his expensive hooded top. "Get out! Now! I can't take this any more."

"Fuck off." He tried to wriggle free of my grasp on his hood. "Get the fuck off my jacket you slag."

"I mean it Tom," I shrieked breathlessly. "I want you out of this house till you've calmed down. I don't have to put up with this."

I retreated into the kitchen to get away from him.

"You either give me money or I'm going to sell summat," he hollered after me.

"Try it mate." I tried to make my tone nonchalant. "I'll ring the police."

"You'd better say goodbye to the TV!" He yanked the plug out of the wall.

"Tom, stop this or I'm ringing Martin!" I flounced back into the living room.

"I'll fucking smash the house up!" No sooner had the words escaped him before he began kicking and fisting the wall in the living room, quickly resulting in two gaping holes in the plaster."

Grabbing my phone, I dialled 999.

"You fucking bitch!" He lunged at my phone. "You're not getting me locked up!"

"Watch me!"

He grabbed his coat and trainers as I was connected.

"Police please." This was unreal. *I was ringing the police because I was scared of my own son!* I fought to regain my breath and my heart felt like it was thudding in my ears. Tom was still in the house as my call was connected. I decided to proceed with it.

"My son's being verbally abusive and threatening. He's booting my walls in!" I garbled at the operator.

"What you fucking lying for!"

He left before the police arrived. Thankfully, they didn't treat me like a timewaster as I had feared.

"What is it you want us to do?" the policewoman asked gently, after I had relayed what had happened.

"I think the fact that I've rung you has shown him I mean business. But I guess I'd like you to give him a warning."

"Would you be willing to go to court and testify against him?"

I laughed sarcastically through my tears. "Court. They won't do a thing. They never do."

"I know," she agreed. "It frustrates us too. Anyway it's your call. We can put a warrant out for him but you have to be willing to follow it through."

I hesitated. "This time I think I'll leave it but if there's a next time I'll follow it up, all the way."

"You won't get this choice again. I have to make you aware of that. I know he's your son but we're classing this as a domestic abuse incident." Her words reverberated in my ears as she made several jottings in her 'pocketbook.'

"Next time, we can do what's known as a 'victimless prosecution.' Also, you need to know that if he'd still been in the house when we got here, we'd have arrested him. It would have been taken it out of your hands."

I understood perfectly. They left soon after, promising me the whole incident was 'on record' and I could use it against Tom should anything else occur.

I rang Martin.

"He's out! He's out!" was the only response he could muster to my frantic wittering. Quickly, I ended the 'conversation' before telephoning Tom's youth offending worker.

"I can't cope any more," I wept down the phone. "Martin wants to chuck him out *now*. So do I, to be honest, but obviously I won't."

"Why not? He *is* actually old enough now. I know he'd have to move into a hostel but only for a month or so before something more secure was sorted."

"There must be an alternative."

"Sarah, I doubt he'll get offered a council flat. Not for years." She fell silent for a moment. "I can arrange for our housing officer to do a home visit though. She knows of one or two supported housing schemes, so might have a few suggestions. If you're willing to *officially* threaten him with homelessness, I think he'd fulfil their criteria."

Hope began to flood into me like torrential rain into a water butt. "I think it's the only way forward. Is there any way you can sort me an appointment with her? If I know there's movement with getting him housed and supported, I'll be strong enough to hang in here a bit longer."

"Well, he certainly ticks all the boxes. Young person. Family breakdown. Threatened with homelessness. Substance misuse. Offending behaviour."

It was a miserable list but at that moment it was lifesaving debris in a turbulent ocean. Something to cling onto.

"Sarah, I want him out you know." Martin surveyed the holes in the wall then turned to me. "You hold the key. I can't throw him out. You're his mother. It's your call."

"I'm onto it." I then relayed the information about the housing schemes.

"That could drag on for bloody months." He slapped the palm of his hand against his leg. "How much longer can we go on like this? We can't have a holiday. We can't trust him with the house or even a key to the house. Everything has to be locked away from him." His tone heightened as he reeled off the situation. "He won't change, you know. Things are getting worse as far as I'm concerned."

"I know. But I'm going to do everything I can to get it

sorted."

"But why should *I* have to keep living like it?" He threw his arms into the air. "Why should Alex? Even Peter doesn't want to know. And he's his *father.* So why the hell should I?"

"Cos you've been here since he was this big." I gestured by flattening the palm of my hand down beside my knee. "I don't believe you can chuck him out with nowhere to go, any more than I can."

"Watch me." He folded his arms and surveyed me with an air of defiance.

"Martin, he might leave for a couple of days but then what?" I held my hands out in question. "He'd be back: begging, pleading. Could you lie in bed at night, listening to him at the door, hammering on it, shouting that he's nowhere to sleep and feeling hungry?"

"No." He admitted after a few moments thought.

"Which is why we've *got* to do this properly. We need to arrange a suitable flat where he'll have support with everything. He'll get help with his drugs problems too."

It was only me preventing him being thrown out. Martin did not want him there. The neighbours didn't. Alex certainly didn't. Neither did I, but I had to do what was right.

Within days, we had another visit from the police. Martin dealt with it. I was grateful I was out. He rang me after they had gone.

"The police have just been," he informed me, wearily.

"Oh no! Hang on. I'm driving. Let me put you on speakerphone."

Hurriedly, I clipped the phone on the dashboard and awaited further information.

"There was two of them." As I manoeuvred the car around a bend, I strained to hear what he was saying. Alex sat bolt upright in the passenger seat, his eyes gleaming in anticipation of what his stupid brother might have done this time.

"He hasn't actually done anything," Martin explained. "They just wanted a word about him and this anti-social contract thing."

"They've already written to me about it." My relief was palpable at the realisation that he had not actually *done* anything.

"I know. But they're saying things haven't improved. And they're right, aren't they? Anyway, they had a sheet with about ten photos on. There was a picture of Tom among them and I recognised about six of the others."

"So?"

"They're the lads they're going to force out of the area apparently. They don't care how they do it but have said enough is enough. The visit was to warn us of what's going to happen."

"That's noble of them. Martin, I just can't handle any more of this shit." I pulled over in order to continue the conversation so Alex could only hear one side of it.

"They asked if we could contact the housing association about being re-housed," Martin went on. "Or if we've any family we could stay with."

"I told them we're not going anywhere; we've done nothing wrong, and shouldn't have to lose our home because of Tom. One of them warned we won't have a choice soon."

"What're we going to do?"

"Look I don't know how. But we're going to *have* to get Tom out. If we don't, he's going to take us *all* down with him." Martin's voice was firm and I knew he was right. "We'll be in a hostel or something before we know it, if we don't get this mess sorted. Can't you have another word with his dad? See if he'll take him in."

"No point. I already know what response I'll get. Look he's sixteen now. Hopefully one of
these supported housing schemes will come to something."

"We haven't got time for all that. Whilst he's still living here, he's got to change. We're going to lose everything if he doesn't."

"How often have we tried talking to him!' Martin, we could physically lock him in his room and he'd just break out of the window! We've no say over anything he does!"

"What's up Mummy?" Alex's voice was small beside me.

"Nothing sweetheart. Don't you worry about anything." I rested a reassuring hand on his knee. "Mummy will get it all sorted, I promise."

"One of them noticed the holes in the wall as well." Martin continued.

"What did you say?"

"The truth. I think she's going to tell the housing though. She mentioned criminal damage."

"Look we'll fight this." From nowhere, a sense of fight emerged. "All the way. There's *no way* we're getting thrown out. I'll get a solicitor involved if I have to. We have rights. We've done nothing wrong."

"We're responsible for everyone in our house. That's what they're saying. If Tom's out of control, we're liable."

"That's just it. When hasn't he been out of control?"

Holding On

Tom *didn't* get offered a place at art college. He had become so accustomed to a one-to-one forum where he was able to discuss his issues, that unfortunately, he had not made this distinction when being interviewed by the college.

He had disclosed all his drugs problems to his interviewer whose response had been scepticism as to whether he would possess the concentration or commitment required to succeed at the course.

His future and where he could possibly be heading was a source of incessant worry for me. As the days wore on, Tom was increasingly directionless and unoccupied.

Each morning, before leaving for work, I would stow away my computer and Alex's games console. Frequently we would return home to find his friends loitering around the house, usually fed and watered at our expense. I felt like running away and leaving them all to it. I never knew what state things were going to be in when I returned. My home was beyond my control. These fears were heightened by the knowledge that the neighbours were documenting everything. All my hopes were pinned upon the forthcoming appointment with the housing officer.

*　*　*

Despite his promises, Tom did not return home at the appointed time.

"I can't proceed without him here," the woman explained as she sipped her tea. "There are various forms he needs to sign."

"Can't I just do it for him?"

She shook her head. "We can discuss his support needs and what accommodation is available but I can't actually commit him to anything without meeting him."

"I understand." I cast another cursory glance out of the window and along the street.

"So, are we looking at emergency accommodation?" She tugged some leaflets from her bag. "Do you require him out immediately?"

I recoiled in shame. *What an awful situation!* "No, not immediately, I want to hang in there and make sure he's alright. He's still so young, particularly emotionally." The woman scribbled away as I spoke. "I want him to have support with his drugs and offending issues. Oh, and budgeting and living skills and all that kind of thing. Having said that, I won't turn my back once he's in his own place. I'll still be keep an eye on him and will be there for him."

"Well that's a real positive for him." Stopping her writing, she looked at me.

"Really?"

"You'd be surprised how many parents of the kids I deal with; are booted out and just left to fend for themselves."

"I'm not kicking him out. But I need to get something in place before we all lose our home, and I lose my mind!"

She laughed slightly. "I've been briefed by Tom's youth offending worker. It sounds as though things have been rough. She says you've done as much as you can."

I nodded, feeling grateful for this acknowledgement. "Really the only thing standing in the way of him needing emergency accommodation right now, is me. If it was up to my husband, Tom's stepdad, he'd be out straightaway."

Just then Tom walked or should I say, stumbled, in. At first, I was dismayed to realise he was out of his mind and hoped the housing woman wouldn't notice. However, there was no masking his state when he attempted to string a sentence together. Thankfully, he wasn't too stoned to sign his name several times on the paperwork.

The situation began to look promising. He was to be referred for a flat where he would have an allocated support worker. Help would be given with benefits, leisure time usage, budgeting and cooking. Due to his history of drug taking and offending, he was definitely eligible. Although he was stupid enough to think there was a benefit in lying about it all.

"I don't touch cannabis anymore," he asserted when the housing worker questioned him about his history of drug use.

"Tom you're stoned now!"

"Shut the fuck up!" He accepted one of the forms to sign.

"Tom don't talk to your mum like that." She passed him her pen. "Not in front of me please. It's awful."

"Well she don't know shit." His voice slurred as he spoke. "She just thinks she does."

"How long are we talking before things start moving?" This was the question. *How long would I have to wait until I could have some sort of normal home?* Not having to lock everything away and lug my handbag around with me. Not to be abused and sworn at on a daily basis. To be able to go to bed, knowing I would not be disturbed at any time; either by Tom returning at all hours, or his associates, causing trouble outside the house."

"Probably just a couple of months." She began sweeping her paperwork into a pile.

"Really?" My voice conveyed surprise yet what I felt was shock.....and an overwhelming sense of guilt.

"Can you can hang in there?" she smiled sympathetically as she nodded towards the holes in the walls.

"I've hung in this long," I sighed as I stood up. "A couple more months won't kill me, I hope!"

"I'll get the referrals in straight away." She clicked the forms inside her bag.

"I'm sorry about the state he was in," I felt ashamed of him as I showed her out.

"Don't worry, I've seen worse!"

After she had gone, I descended onto the bottom step of the staircase, relief washing over me at the progress that had been made.

This was swiftly overshadowed by more guilt. Tom was not even seventeen, yet I was forcing him to leave home. It shouldn't have been this way. I would worry about him endlessly after his departure and would have to restrain myself from checking up on him morning, noon and night.

For all our sakes though, the time was coming where I knew I was going to *have* to let him go. It was time to allow him to sink or swim. Whatever was coming was out of my hands.

Hanging in There

The summer holidays could not arrive soon enough, so I would be off work for six weeks and could try to reclaim control over my house.

One night I lay in bed grimacing as I was woken by a motorbike. It thundered up and down, outside our house for about ten minutes. *The whole street must have been woken!*

It was 2:03. After several more minutes the bike began sounding its horn. Exhausted from the hectic day I had endured before, I felt paralysed.

Then I heard Tom's voice permeating the night air from his bedroom window. "Gimme a minute."

After clattering around his room for several moments, he descended the stairs then climbed out of the living room window. Wide awake now, I listened as the deafening engine roared again, before commencing its exit from the street. Gradually it became remote. Its drone resonated inside my shattered mind. *What if Tom wasn't wearing a helmet?* My eyes flickered back open in the darkness, my maternal urge overshadowing my exhaustion.

I prayed they would be stopped by police. I lay for ages, gazing into the void of the night, still hearing the motorbike's engine inside my head until after 4 am. I was going to struggle getting up for work at six, yet the more I worried about this, the more sleepless I became.

Finally I must have dropped off because I can recall my irritation when Martin nudged me in the ribs at 4.35 to inform me that Tom was re-entering our home through the living room window. Relieved as I was, I still felt extreme anger as I heard him clattering about in the kitchen downstairs, preparing himself some food.

Less than two hours later, I dragged myself out of bed, furiously noticing he had pulled the entire curtain rail out of the plaster during either his exit or entrance through the window. Rage coursed through my body along with the coffee I sipped. Every measure would need to be employed to keep me awake at work! However, I battled with a migraine all day.

I should have looked forward to finishing work for the day, but home did not feel like home anymore. As I neared the street, the usual tug of dread could be felt, in the depths of my stomach, as I anticipated who might be loitering around; the state of the house and the mood Tom might be in.

"What was I supposed to do all day without any bloody money?" he scowled at me from the armchair as I crept in, laden with bags. Again, I felt like blubbing as I glanced around. I could not go on much longer. The kitchen was splattered with fat from his culinary attempts. Four pints of milk had been guzzled. Wrappers and half eaten food were strewn everywhere and he was as usual, wearing Martin's socks.

What may sound trivial to others was beginning to irk me beyond belief. Even though he had in excess of twenty pairs of socks, he would still help himself to whatever he wanted, regardless of whether it belonged to someone else.

I scrabbled about in my purse before thrusting a five pound note at him.

"Is that it?" He inspected the note as though it was a dead mouse.

"We have this conversation nearly every day Tom," I began shuffling towards the kitchen with my shopping. "I shouldn't give you anything. You cause me nothing but heartache, you don't lift a finger in the house and to be honest you're old enough to be getting a job at the weekend."

"Yeah, right." Stuffing the note into his pocket, he then set about getting ready to go out. This consisted of him cramming his pockets with food, coating gel on his hair and spraying Lynx on himself with such voracity that he would be smelt streets away!

Eventually a banged door indicated his departure. He was apparently not blessed with social niceties, such as saying *bye mum, see you later!*

As was often the case, I locked the house up that night unaware of whether Tom would be back or not. Sleep found Martin easily; this was never the case with me! It was a luxury I had learned to forsake long before. And with good reason.

It was a warm night as I lay with the window ajar. In the distance I began to hear shouting. And lots of it. Somebody was obviously having an altercation. The voices grew closer. There seemed to be a whole gang of them.

"Gerroff me!" By now whatever was going on had typically found its way to the end of my street. I could see it all from my window. Some sort of fight. Furious, heightened voices which were descending into violence. There was someone beneath that lot. There were about ten lads; it looked like a rugby scrum. Only this was ten onto one. And that *one*, I realised in horror, was Tom. On autopilot I fired myself down the stairs and out into the street.

"Get off him!" I hurtled towards them all. "Leave him alone!" Several of them startled as they surveyed me, pyjama clad. The neighbours must have got tired of seeing me running wildly into the street, in my nightwear, trying to avert some crisis or other! I stood, watching defiantly until one by one they released their grip upon him.

"Woman beater!" mocked one, releasing Tom but shoving him as he did. "You'll keep." Tom floundered towards me, his lip bloodied and eye blackened. The gang of boys diffused.

"Are you OK?" I caught him by the arm to steady him. "Why've they done this to you?"

"Just leave it mum." He tried to tug his arm away.

"I will *not* leave it. I've a good mind to call the police."

"Then I'll be in even worse shit!" He checked back over his shoulder.

"Why?" Pausing, I studied his face. "What have you done?"

"I haven't done owt, not that *you'll* believe me." He scowled, wincing in pain in the process.

"Sit there." I commanded as we entered the living room. "I'll get something to bathe your face."

"It's fine. I'm OK." But he slumped down anyway.

I returned to the room armed with water and cotton wool. "I want to know why they were after you."

"Some girl's whining I smacked her. She was my girlfriend but not any more. I didn't though, honest mum." Beseechingly, he stared at me as I wrung water out of the cotton wool. "I just dumped her and she's upset so she's making up lies."

"Are you sure?"

"See, I knew you wouldn't believe me. You never do!"

"Alright Tom, calm down!" I dabbed at his eye.

"Ouch!"

"Tom if you *did* hit her, tell me."

"I didn't. Not that they'll take any notice. It was her brother who organised that lot." He gestured towards the window. "They'll be waiting for me every night from now on."

Under his injuries, he looked defeated and weary. Inwardly, I prayed that we soon had an alternative for him. For his own sake as much as anybody else's he needed to get out of the area. A new start was essential.

The Supported Housing Project

August 2010 (16 years, 8 months)

"How long's it likely to take?"

The ample woman handed Tom the form to sign. "It could be a month." Her jowls wobbled with her words. "It could be a year. It all depends on the turnover of residents. I have to say though....." She glanced down at one of the newly completed forms. "He'll be getting the highest priority awarded."

"Will he?"

"Yes." Her cigarette-affected voice rasped as she replied. "He's threatened with homelessness and because of his age, it shouldn't be that long. We usually prioritise the referrals we get from the youth offending housing worker."

The word *homelessness* deeply pierced my conscience.

"I reckon I'd be alright here." Tom leaned back in his chair, clasping his hands behind his head as he surveyed the grounds of the housing complex.

I had been pleasantly surprised by the surroundings. The gardens were carefully landscaped, full of greenery and areas in which to sit. Ironically, the accommodation had echoes of the chalets we had previously holidayed in.

"Would you like to have a look at one of the flats?" the lady offered, following Tom's gaze.

"Please!" Tom and I chorused, rising to our feet.

The flat had been freshly painted in magnolia. The wood-effect linoleum on the floor looked new. It contained everything he would need; cooker, fridge, bed, sofa; even curtains.

"You'd have a support worker allocated," advised the woman, watching as we inspected our surroundings. "They'd have a meeting with you as soon as you moved in to see what you'd need help with."

"Everything!" I verified, stopping my inspection and turning to her. "Cooking, cleaning, budgeting, shopping, he hasn't a clue!"

"Well he is young." As he opened and closed kitchen cupboards, she studied him. I could only imagine what must be going through her head about us.

During the interview, Tom had admitted to having a *slight* cannabis problem and to *occasionally* going off the rails when he was *younger;* also having previously been in trouble with the police. *But that was all behind him now.* He had said as much. I had resisted the urge to complicate matters and had not contradicted the information he had given. *What would be the point?* It might make the difference between him being accepted onto the waiting list, or not.

Throughout the interview, he had been uncharacteristically pleasant and well-spoken. The woman must have been wondering what on earth had gone sour within our family for me to want him re-housed at such a vulnerable age.

I no longer wanted to elaborate on the details though. Things just had to move forward. I was sick of having to justify myself, exhausted of going over and over the same background details and reasons for things. There was no point anymore in dealing with things in any other way.

His dad and Elizabeth were no longer able to provide any 'respite,' our reputation lay in shreds where we were living and we were all facing losing our home. Unfortunately the situation had come to this; it was either a case of *him* needing accommodation, or *all* of us.

Tom was incredibly upbeat as we left the supported housing complex and returned to the car. "I liked it there mum. I hope they give me a flat." I nodded, guilt-infested. This was not really what I wanted. It was eating me. But I was clueless as to what else to do.

"Will you drop me off at my mates?" His tone was far more amenable than usual.

The remainder of the brief journey continued in silence. When he got out of the car, he did not even besiege me for money! His six foot form strode away before waving back at me! If I hadn't already been sitting, I think I would have wobbled over!

Momentarily, I closed my eyes, trying to make sense of the turmoil swirling around within me. Slipping the car into gear, I set off again. But once around the corner, I parked up and dissolved into tears.

The ringing of my mobile sliced into my depleted mood. It was his youth offending worker, the lady who had initially referred him for the housing assessment.

"How's it all going?"

"Ok." I dabbed my eyes on my sleeve as I tried to steady my voice. "We've just been to look at *Maple Court*."

"Oh, the supported housing unit. Yes, it's not too bad there. He should be OK."

"I know. It's just he's so young." A fresh tide of sorrow engulfed me. "I'm sure the woman who interviewed him was judging me, thinking, *why are you kicking your son out?*" I choked a sob down.

"She won't have been, don't worry. They're aware that young people referred there have a variety of issues. In fact she was probably shocked that he was accompanied by his mother for the interview. Most young people in there are alone in life."

Tears were cascading from my eyes again. Holding the phone away from my face, I sniffed.

"Sarah, are you OK?"

"Not really. I just feel so guilty." My voice wobbled, uncontrollably. Damm, she would know I was crying now!

"You've nothing to feel guilty about. You've been through a hell of a time with Tom. You've got to let him go now. I'm not saying it'll be easy, but maybe you're doing him the biggest favour you possibly could."

"I don't see how."

"What chance does he have if he stays where he is? Amongst the others, amongst the drugs? What chance do any of you have? You've told me yourself you'll all be kicked out. Sarah, I think you've done as much as you can."

"It's not as if I'm going to turn my back at him." The lump in my throat felt like a melon. "I'll still be helping him out and keeping watch over him." I shielded my face from a woman who strolled past my car, peering at me curiously.

"I know that. You won't suddenly stop being his mum just because he's not living with you."

"I just wish I didn't feel so awful." I fished around in my bag for a tissue.

"You're bound to. It's a massive step. But with a bit of luck, it'll all turn out OK. It's up to Tom. He's not a little boy any more."

"I know," I sniffed, wiping my eyes. "I suppose I was out on my own at his age and managed. And I didn't have *anyone* to lean on."

The Phone Call

It was a beautiful Sunday morning. I sat, sprawled amongst the chaos I had caused in Alex's bedroom. Clothes, books, outgrown toys, bits of things; we were having a clear out.

Alex had initially assisted but swiftly become bored and gone out to play football. In the distance I could hear him, shrieking and yelling with his friends.

From the next room, our bedroom, I listened to the rhythmic strokes of the paint roller as Martin applied the lovely lilac paint I had chosen to our bedroom wall. Lilac, in the hope of creating a relaxing ambience! *Odour free*, it had claimed. But the entire house reeked of paint. It was not an unpleasant smell though. Things smelt transformed and clean.

Tom, who had not graced us with his presence until after three in the morning, still slept. I glanced out of Alex's window at the cloudless blue sky beyond. What a waste of life. It was nearly midday. How could he still be sleeping? My thoughts were interrupted by the ringing of my mobile phone.

"Can I speak to Tom please?" The voice sounded official. Strange that; on a Sunday morning.

"He's asleep, I'm afraid. Can I help at all?"

"Are you his mum?"

"Yes." *Oh God, please don't say he's in trouble again!*

"It's Linda, calling from Maple Court; he attended an interview last week."

"Yes, that's right." *I hoped there wasn't a problem with his application.*

"I'm sorry to bother you on a Sunday but we've a vacant flat that we'd like to offer him."

I couldn't speak. I needed a moment to process her words.

"Are you there?"

"Yes. Sorry." I sank back against the boxes that surrounded me. "You've got an empty flat?"

"That's right. But we need to know *now* whether he wants to accept it. And for Housing Benefit purposes, he'd need to have it signed up by tomorrow."

"Tomorrow?" I gulped.

"Yes, would that be a problem?"

"N, no, I shouldn't think so." The 'melon' abruptly returned to my throat. "When would he move in?"

"Well, we can complete the signing up process at five o'clock tomorrow, which gives us chance to do our checks on the flat during the day. So he can move in tomorrow night."

"That soon?" I felt dizzy.

"I thought that's what he wanted?"

"It is." Tears warmed my eyes. "It's just a bit of a shock. Sorry."

"Should I go ahead and make the appointment for him," she bristled.

"Yes, I think so."

"Do you need to check with him first?"

"No, I know it's what he wants."

"Right. Good. We'll see you tomorrow at five then. He'll need evidence of his identity and his national insurance number."

After the conversation had ended, I continued to sit amidst the mess I had created. I am not sure how long I sat there. The room appeared to swim around me as I tried to focus my jangling thoughts.

Finally, I went to enlighten Martin. Perching on the edge of our bed, I watched him roller the paint onto the wall for a moment.

"Nice colour," I remarked, absently, trying to hold the heaviness out of my voice. You're doing a good job."

"Who was on the phone?"

"Maple Court."

"The place you had the appointment at?" Without looking at me, he continued to roller, not noticing tears spilling down my cheeks.

"That's the one."

"What did they want?"

"To offer Tom a flat." The words left me slowly. I could hardly believe I had uttered them.

"WHAT?" Martin swung around to face me. "You're joking. This soon? When?"

"Tomorrow."

"Tomorrow!" He dropped the paint roller in its tray. "You mean he's actually going to be moving out *tomorrow*?" He made no effort to disguise the excitement in his voice.

"That's what I said." I stared blankly at the floor.

"Why are you crying?" He shook his head at me. "You should be pleased!"

"*Pleased?* Don't be ridiculous. He's my son." I drifted out of the room and downstairs before trying to distract myself in the kitchen. Martin quickly followed.

"Sarah get a grip, for God's sake." He reached for my arm. "This is what we've all needed for a long time, Tom included."

I continued to stack the dishwasher so I didn't have to look at him. The level of my anguish had taken me by surprise. Had I allowed the stray tears to become sobs, they may never have stopped. Suddenly, Tom felt like my defenceless child again and I was no longer certain I felt prepared to let him go. Suddenly, I had visions of my tiny blonde boy, and flashes in my mind of pulling him back from the road or preventing him from climbing too high.

Martin caught my elbow and forced me to face him. His voice became gentler when he realised how affected I was.

"Can you imagine what'll happen if we don't take this chance?" He caught my chin in his hand. "We'll all be booted out of this house within a few months. Think of it Sarah. Think of what we've been through. But most of all; think of Alex!" His voice had a pleading edge to it.

I knew this was it. There was no way we could go back on things now.

"I'm going to take the dog out for a bit." I yanked the lead from its hook. "I need to clear my head."

I made the short journey to the next village, tears rolling down my face as I listened to the ebb and flow of the engine. I stopped at the supermarket to buy meat for Sunday dinner. *What if this was the last time he wanted to eat his Sunday dinner with us?*

It was one of those scorching, summery days where most people feel ecstatic to be alive. I approached the checkout, noticing that people were buying boxes of lager, chicken drumsticks and other barbecue paraphernalia. There was an energized undercurrent as children queued with their parents, eagerly anticipating a fun family afternoon.

"Is that all you've got love?" A woman's voice distracted me. "You might as well go before us."

"Thanks." I slapped the lone piece of silverside onto the conveyer belt. As I waited for it to be scanned, I caught sight of a tiny boy in the woman's trolley. My breath caught in my throat as I observed the shafts of sunlight refracting back from his white-blonde hair. For an instant it was though a young Tom had come back, to taunt me, to portray the enormity of the situation which was now presenting itself.

The dog and I trudged around the adjacent park for what seemed like an eternity. The idea had been to try and collect my thoughts a little and give myself a bit of a talking to, but I was enveloped by a numb, foggy feeling. Though one foot went in front of the other, I felt incomplete. Nothing would ever be the same again. With every family I saw, every mother with her son, my depression deepened. I hated myself. *How could I be doing this to my sixteen-year-old?*

Tom was just stirring when I arrived home. His mood seemed as dark as ever as he crashed around the kitchen. I took a deep breath.

"Maple Court have rung." I pulled a pan from the cupboard. "You know, the place where you saw a flat last week?"

"Oh yeah?"

"They've got a flat for you." I began to unwrap the beef. "They want you to move in tomorrow." I studied his reaction. A grin that appeared to be a combination of relief and gratitude stretched across his face.

"You're kidding! Honest?"

"Yep." I dropped the beef in the pan with a thud. "How do you feel about it?"

"It's the bizz, I can't believe it." Leaning against the fridge door, he was seemingly overcome. "But what'll I do for money?"

"We'll get all that sorted out." I threw the pan into the oven. "Do you definitely want to go? Cos you don't have to, you know."

"Sarah." Martin jumped up from his chair. "We all know it's for the best."

"I know." I lowered my eyes so neither of them would notice see the fresh batch of tears that were bubbling up. I busied myself in folding tea towels that were already folded. "I suppose we'd better get you sorted then."

"Shall I start packing? Have you got any boxes or owt?"

Without waiting for an answer, he sped upstairs. Sliding floorwards against the kitchen cupboard, I sobbed into my hands.

"It's the end of an era," announced Martin, rubbing his hands together. "This is it. He's leaving home."

"He's too young!" I wailed, staring at the checked pattern on the lino.

"Pull yourself together, for God's sake." He felt in his pockets for his wallet. "I'm going for a pint to celebrate."

"You're all heart, aren't you?"

For much of the day, I continued in the same vein. I was unable to stop crying but somehow managed to conceal from Tom just how distressed I was. I certainly could never have predicted the extent to which the offer of the flat would upset me.

"Just because you're moving out, it doesn't mean you're on your own." I had pulled myself together adequately enough to give Tom a 'pep-talk' as I ironed. I'll still be helping you." The steam curled up towards my face, its warmth providing momentary comfort.

"Yeah, I know."

"This is your big chance." Filling the iron with water, I tried to stop my stressed-out hand from trembling. "It's up to you what you do with your life now."

"Yeah, whatever." He turned the volume up on the TV.

"For goodness sake, don't be having all your mates around. They won't give a toss if you end up losing your flat. They won't think twice about messing everything up for you."

"I know."

"And as for smoking cannabis in there. If you were to get caught, you'd probably get kicked out."

"Alright Mum. Stop going on. You're doing my head in now." His eyes remained fixed to the TV. I continued to iron; slamming it down onto every garment, wishing my misery would evaporate with the steam.

He stayed at home that night. I listened to every creak and cough from his room, knowing I was hearing him in the next room for the last time. It was like a bereavement. I lay, staring into the darkness, waiting for tears or sleep to come. Tears kept winning the battle. By three o'clock I'd had enough of just lying there and went downstairs. The early summer sun rose, marking the dawn of the final day I would have my son at home. Still sobbing, I drifted off to sleep on the sofa.

Moving On

"I've packed me stuff mum." Tom arrived at the bottom of the stairs, laden with bags. "It's all there." His mood had lifted enormously since the flat had been offered.

"Right." My heart felt like rock as I observed his new-found cheeriness. "I'll get you plates, towels and stuff like that packed. I'm not sure what's in the flat already but you'll want stuff of your own." I began tugging various items from the kitchen cupboards.

"What time do I need to be back here?" He leant down to fasten his trainers.

"Where are you off?"

"Just round and about."

"Tom, don't be telling people where the flat is." I stacked several plates into a box. "It's going to be your place, *yours* and no one else's."

"I know."

It's where you can come and go, lock your door behind you and do whatever you want." I watched him as he swapped feet to tie his other lace. "Your space. Your sanctuary."

"All right Mum, you're going on again." He rose to his feet.

"I'm saying all this cos your so-called mates will have no qualms about seeing you booted out of there." I was aware that I was following him as I rattled on. He dragged his hooded top from the coat hooks. "This is a new beginning for you, an opportunity for you to rid yourself of the idiots around here. You'll have me around to help you. And support workers. Use them. Make the most of them."

"I'm off anyway. Can I have some money?"

For the first time since I'd woke up on the sofa, I wept again as I observed his lanky frame strut off down the street. As I surveyed the pile of bags and boxes, I wondered if I'd ever stop.

Part of me wanted to get the move over and done with, but this wrestled with the other part of me that wanted to put all his belongings back in his room, and call Maple Court to tell them he had changed his mind. Deep down, however, I knew this was not an option.

The day ticked by like any other. Trying to keep myself occupied was difficult as I was struggling to focus on anything. Tom was unusually punctual and arrived home for the final time at the prearranged time of 4.00 pm. Martin helped him load up my car with his belongings. I couldn't bear to.

We travelled in silence, save for the occasional chatter from Tom. It was as though he had been given a personality transplant.

Maple Court was bathed in sunshine when we arrived; one or two of the residents ambled around in the grounds. Tom jumped out of the car and swaggered into the reception area as though he owned the place. I crept in behind him, not daring to meet anyone's gaze with my downcast, red-rimmed eyes.

"If you'd just like to have a seat in there." The woman who had previously interviewed Tom beckoned us into a side room, the flesh on the tops of her arms swaying with the force of the movement. Moments later she joined us, accompanied by a man, Carl, who was to be Tom's housing support worker.

"Right Tom. This is a copy of your tenancy agreement." The paper crackled as she passed it to him. "If you could just sign there."

"This is your application for Housing Benefit. You need to sign it there and there." She pointed, appropriately.

I listened peripherally as the formalities took place. It felt like a dream. And I was certain that the woman kept looking at me, wondering what sort of a mother I must be to be allowing my son to leave home at sixteen.

Martin and Alex waited in the car. They were to be given the nod when the official stuff had taken place in order that they could begin carting everything in.

I trudged behind the party of three to be shown the flat. Electric meter, post, laundry, etc, etc. Tom did not seem to be listening but displayed a euphoric expression. Especially when handed his key.

"There's a £5 charge if you lose it," advised the woman in a mock-stern tone.

Between us, it did not take long to unload his belongings.

"You've got some sorting out to do tonight Tom." I flicked my eyes around the flat, breathing in the scent of fresh paint and new linoleum.

"I'll tell you something Tom, this isn't bad," Martin called from the kitchen as he opened and closed doors. "You've got a real chance here. Make sure you don't blow it."

A trip around the supermarket was necessary, so we could at least leave him with full cupboards and a well-stocked fridge.

"I can see I've got a lot to teach you about shopping!" I remarked as he tried to sling in whatever took his fancy without even glancing at the price.

As we drove back to the flat, I further eased my conscience by buying him cigarettes and crediting his phone. Then we took him and Alex for tea. I was too churned up to eat anything. Eventually, the inevitable had to take place. We had to drop him off.

"I'll ring you in the morning," I promised, my voice wobbling uncontrollably. "We'll leave you alone now and let you get settled."

"OK Mum." For a moment I thought he was going to hug me. Fleetingly, the wall between us crumbled. I hugged him instead.

"You'll be OK won't you?" I battled to hold back the tears. "I do love you, you know. Don't ever forget that."

He didn't answer but for once, just hugged me back.

"Come on Sarah. Let's leave him to it. He looks done in." Martin's voice came quietly from the doorway.

"I'm off home to get a glass of wine." I stood back from him. "Ring me if you need anything. Anything at all."

"Is he staying there for ever Mummy?" Alex whispered from behind me as I got into the car.

"We'll just have to see." The urge to return to the flat and retrieve him was overwhelming.

"Are you OK Mummy?"

"I'll be fine." I didn't turn to look at him but was warmed by his concern. We were all exhausted and I needed to pull myself back together. Poor Alex had hardly had any attention from me for two days. But he would now have me all to himself. Not that I had stopped being Tom's Mum. In fact, I was feeling a maternal tug towards him more powerfully than I had in years.

Alex quickly got into his pyjamas when we arrived home.

"Come and tuck me in Mummy." His little arms wrapped around my neck more tightly than usual. I managed to make it out of his room before the tears surged again.

"I'm taking the dog onto the field," I announced to Martin.

"Shall I come with you?" The field overlooked our house. I poured myself a large glass of wine to carry over with me.

"No. I could do with a bit of time on my own. I won't be long."

I sprawled on the grass, as the dog bounced around me, staring over at the stillness of my house, aglow in the late sunset. The street was motionless and a solitary bird sang, its tune carried around by the feeble breeze.

Before long, sobs ceased to wrack my body. As the sun sank further behind the house, I shivered in the sudden chill of the air. I leaned forward and hugged my knees towards me, enjoying the momentary warmth they provided.

A picture of my son crept back into my mind as I imagined him in his flat amongst his belongings. For a moment I ached and prayed with all my heart he would be OK. At least he was happy, of that; I was sure. For now, anyway. That was all I had ever wanted for him; happiness.

As the sky grew darker, I noticed a large star. It glowed in front of me, its clarity protruding amongst the others. When I was young, my grandma had told me to always wish on the first star I saw at night. But she told me never to speak my wish out loud or it would not come true. For several minutes, I gazed at the star before closing my eyes to wish. Like I had never wished before.

An overwhelming sense of peace crept around me as a single tear slid down my cheek.

In Mourning

I glance at the boy from over the street
who outwardly has the world at his feet;
he easily slings his bag on his back
containing his schoolbooks; the ones that you lack.

I observe a boy; with his dog he strides out
"Why isn't he like you?" I feel I could shout;
content with his life as his dog leaps around,
not needing and craving the props that you've found.

Another boy passes; errands on a list,
tears well inside for the boy that I've missed
who cares for his mother and eases her load
whilst you choose to hurtle far down the wrong road.

My attentions diverted by some raucous noise,
a ball's kicked about by a huddle of boys;
their carefree laughter rings out as they run,
that's where you should be, fusing in fun.

A shriek of his brakes as a boy cycles by,
his bike gives him wings; makes him able to fly;
why, in your life, do you not have that pride?
Your rapid descent makes me sting inside.

I look at these boys, so healthy and strong,
amongst them you'd be, it's where you belong;
weakened and gaunt with pallor so pale,
I'm so scared one day I'll be mourning for real.

Printed in Great Britain
by Amazon